# MARGARET OVERTON

# HOPE FOR A COOL PILLOW

Outpost19 | San Francisco
outpost19.com

Overton, Margaret
        Hope For a Cool Pillow / Margaret Overton
        ISBN 9781937402907 (pbk)

Library of Congress Control Number: 2015919193

Cover art by Alex Nowik

OUTPOST19

ORIGINAL
PROVOCATIVE
READING

# HOPE FOR A
# COOL PILLOW

For Larry

## Author's Note

This book is an exploration of end-of-life care based on my experiences as a daughter and as a physician. It recounts the gradual evolution of a viewpoint regarding an important and complex issue. All patient information has been altered to protect individual identities and respect privacy.

The story does not follow a traditional chronological course; rather it follows the path I took in figuring it out. Which means I wrote it slightly backwards, looping about, side to side, and with the considerable use of retrospect. Things rarely work out as we plan; but without a plan, where would we be?

—*Margaret Overton*

# PART ONE

# One

On the first day of my first clinical rotation in the third year of medical school, I was assigned my first patient. Her name was Esther. An internal medicine resident told me to insert a urinary catheter into Esther, who hadn't peed in a day or so.

Placing the catheter would mark another first. But the problem proved murkier: how to make the transition from a normal social interaction to elbowing apart the knees of a stranger and mucking about in her nether region. The whole concept seemed intrusive, certainly an invasion of her privacy. I hadn't learned the necessary etiquette from gross anatomy, physical diagnosis, or Emily Post. So I called my mother from the nursing station. Her knowledge of decorum was encyclopedic.

"You got me, honey," Mom said. "I can't help you with this one."

Esther was a hundred and two but she looked lovely nonetheless, sitting up straight in her hospital bed, her hair a white halo surrounding a gently grooved face. I recognized the "Q" sign pretty quickly: open mouth slashed at five o'clock by a protruding tongue. I had read that this usually indicated death[i]. I looked for some movement of her chest but it remained perfectly still. Was it possible that the resident might have sent me to place a catheter in a dead person? Apparently it was not only possible.

Scrambled eggs marred Esther's otherwise tidy hospital gown. Someone must have tried to feed her, not noticing she couldn't swallow, not recognizing she had passed.

That morning, on rounds, her geriatrician had announced: "All my patients are *do not resuscitate* unless otherwise specified." So I did not perform CPR.

From the end of the bed I marveled at her quiet aplomb. This is the way to go, I realized. Nobody stomping on your chest, zapping you with excessive voltage, shoving tubes this way and that. A quiet death without fuss or muss. Esther, wearing a pink satin bed jacket, had slipped away peacefully; she had gone doggedly gentle into that good night.

~

My own mother died on September 22nd in the year 2010. I like to think she chose that particular day for reasons of her own—it was the birthday of someone who had displeased her immensely—but death makes it impossible to verify my hypothesis. She was a disciplined and principled woman who stayed true to her beliefs throughout a long life, which ended consistent with her trusted maxim: *enough is enough*. Had there been a coupon for a coffin—and she'd had her wits about her—I think she would have clipped it. I loved her for that and so much more.

The funeral proceedings took place in the traditional Roman Catholic fashion, with a mass and burial on the day following a wake complete with open casket. I used to think the open casket a barbaric tradition that should be consigned to the past, much like bloodletting for consumption or trephination for mental disorders. It seemed a creepy holdover from a different century. When my father died in 1998, he was almost unrecognizable from the ravages of cancer. Something in me—either doctor or ad hoc decorator—wanted to cover it up. I had suggested to Mom that perhaps we close the casket.

"No," she said firmly at the time, "I want to be able to see him just one more day."

I never understood the open casket until Mom died. Then I needed to be with her, to gaze at her face one more day.

Gibbons Funeral Home, the stalwart if temporary mainstay for the recently departed that graces my hometown of Elmhurst, Illinois, had done a terrific job preparing her hair and make-up. Mom didn't look a day over eighty. My sisters Erica, Beth, Bonnie and I had chosen a suit she'd particularly liked, one that complemented her coloring. We added a cheerful scarf that I had bought her. We picked out her favorite rosary and a pair of coordinating earrings. She looked good, if not well. She certainly did not seem ninety-three. My sisters and I felt confident that Mom would have been thrilled with her posthumous appearance. I'd never given too much thought to cosmetizing, which is the art of making the dead appear better than dead, almost alive really, just kind of still. Or perhaps I'd thought of it in terms of outcome, not in terms of process. It must be a difficult profession, certainly not for everyone. I don't think I'd want to do it, but I've learned from experience that I can do just about anything if I have to.

A surprising number of people showed up for the wake and the funeral. When you're ninety-three, you can't expect too many mourners unless you're famous. Most of your contemporaries are long gone. But Mom still had a few friends who paid their respects. Those who couldn't attend had their children come in their stead. Friends of mine, friends of my sisters', even friends of our kids came to say good-bye to our mother, Lydia Overton. She'd left an impression. I'm not sure you can ask for more than that.

The wake was odd in the manner that wakes usually are, but nothing truly weird happened. Not at the wake anyway. Nobody grabbed any dead body parts or fell to the floor in prostration. I've been at wakes where some distant relatives hauled the dead person up and out of the casket, hugged him, and carried on. I've attended wakes where the family hired a professional to wail. That was definitely awkward and personally discomfiting. My family, for certain, doesn't emote much. Our funerals are civil affairs; the weeping is silent, mostly contained. But still, there we were, standing around a dead body in a casket, making polite small talk about this and that and it was unnerving and frankly pretty damn exhausting trying to pretend it was all just normal, not too devastating really. People I hadn't seen in ages—people I didn't even like—came by to say *hello*. Or *good-bye*, as it were. Some hugs and kisses. I kept glancing over my shoulder at Mom.

It would be my last day with her. Forever. I studied her profile surreptitiously in between visits with other mourners. What if I developed facial agnosia and forgot what she looked like once she was buried? How could pictures ever prove adequate? I wasn't ready for this, and yet she was more than ready. And she was so much more than her image, right? How could a two-dimensional figure evoke the full magnitude of the woman? I was glad to have that one extra day. I needed it. But what I really needed was the mom I'd had years before, when both she and her mind were present in the same room at the same time and we could all have a meaningful discussion. That's the woman I wanted, right here and right now. I wanted her laughter and wisdom; I wanted her insight. But those were long gone.

I kneeled in front of the casket and pretended to pray so I didn't have to talk to anyone. I wanted time alone with her. Mom looked the same in repose as she had each day in recent memory—a slight, beneficent smile affixed to her face. The smile was her default setting, placed there more to reassure than to signal underlying happiness or contentment. Dementia misleads you that way. It's the great teaser, using the expression of equanimity to hide the tragedy of a soul's inching disappearance. But in death her dementia kept its distance; the still silence almost allowed me to forget the previous six years. She was, once again, the brilliant mother who'd taught me to read before I started kindergarten. She'd taught me to cook too, not well, unfortunately, but rather to enjoy the science lab of the kitchen, the science of making do with whatever. Together we experimented with Tollhouse cookies, using butter in differing quantities, baking at differing temperatures, then noting the differences in shape and texture of the cookies. How chewy they turned out. We made fudge, divinity and mincemeat pies at Christmas, banana cream pies for birthdays, and apple-crisps in the fall. I stayed in my bedroom emerging only with flesh-colored nose-plugs when she cooked sauerkraut for my father, or split pea soup for the family. I'd hated her vegetable soup, though it smelled terrific. I refused to learn that recipe. What was I thinking? There were other lessons she taught me, like how to take things apart before sending them to the repair shop. *Always turn the power off and then on before you decide something is broken. Check your connections, check your electrical source, your circuit breakers or fuses, and check your wires; learn how to do basic maintenance on all major appliances simply by following the instructions provided in the manuals—that's what they're there for. If the toilet doesn't flush, take off the top and study the mechanism. It's incredibly simple. Replace the flapper if it doesn't seat properly, they're sold at the hardware store, you know. Change your filters; clean the lint trap; let's follow the hot and cold water lines; you have to know your home. Why hire somebody to do what you can do yourself?*

My daughter Ruthann placed a warm hand on my shoulder. I'd been kneeling a long time.

"Do you want to go get something to drink? There's food in the other room." I stood up, my legs stiff and sore. I looked around. More visitors had gathered. I vaguely recognized most. I should say hello, thank them for coming. Mom would have wanted me to be a gracious hostess, on this occasion as on any other.

"I'm going to sit for a while," I said. "Maybe later."

"Are you okay?" she asked and studied my face. I nodded and sank into an upholstered chair.

It wasn't just home maintenance she'd taught me. Mom preached from the practical to the heartfelt: *High heels will ruin your feet; spend money on decent shoes because when your feet hurt, you hurt all over.* Clean underwear went without saying. *Stand up straight, practice yoga, stretch every day. Send thank-you notes and sympathy cards. Put some thought into what you write. Go to wakes; call friends who've lost a loved one, and don't just call the week after the funeral, but keep calling. The second year is harder than the first.* All of life was a lesson and I trotted along at her heels. She made everything interesting, whether it was how to cut and sew a Vogue pattern, how to hit a golf ball on a downhill lie, or how to choose a ripe pineapple. She taught me how to listen, and how to wonder. She taught me how to focus.

It wasn't that I didn't see this coming. I'd seen it coming for a long time. Maybe that was the problem. The long slow decline was over. And now, what should have been relief turned out to feel like nothing of the sort. Why does grief take us by surprise?

She gave birth to me and then instilled me with everything she knew. What's the opposite of unfurl? That's how her life ended. She folded up. I stood and moved into the crowd. I tried to socialize and make everyone feel welcome, just as my mother would have done.

The funeral showcased the Gibbons' family expertise. The Roman Catholic mass, the drive to the cemetery, and the burial all constituted a precise symphony of tradition and symbolism, each movement perfectly executed by a team with longstanding experience and comfort in their roles. We had only to follow their instructions and our dead would be interred. Wear black, remember lipstick, place tissues in your pocket. Make the sign of the cross and mouth the words to the twenty-third psalm. One final day and this strange but comforting ritual would be complete. Her suffering had ended. Long live suffering. And then, as the graveside service concluded and the mourners began to disperse, Mom's caregiver walked over to the casket and gave full, vibrant voice to her grief, a grief that was completely out of tune with our longstanding civility and repression.

Mom's caregiver was Vicki, a sunny and capable woman in her sixties from the Philippines. She lived in during the last year of Mom's life, sleeping on the sofa in the living room, spending twenty-four hours a day, seven days a week with Mom except for a few days a month when one of her sisters would come to relieve her. Vicki cleaned Mom, dressed Mom, fed Mom. She put make-up on Mom and plucked her eyebrows. She sang to her. She watched an amazing amount of television with Mom, and got her hooked on *Dancing with the Stars* and Filipino Karaoke. Vicki's singing voice made my ears bleed, but Mom loved it. And when Mom died, Vicki grieved, not in the tidy and quiet way of our family, but in the loud and messy way of her own.

It was in that awkward moment at the cemetery, a moment of pure finality and utter solitude—after the prayers had been said, when the visitors began ambling back to their cars, when I felt the slim fragments of religious belief slip further away from me—that Vicki draped herself over the casket and howled. Her chest heaved and her unrestrained sobs filled the dry autumn space of St. Mary's Catholic Cemetery, from which I could see, in the distance to the south, my childhood home. Between my old house and my parents' graves lay the Elmhurst College campus, with its grassy playing fields and nondescript dorms. There used to be tennis courts dividing the graves from the fields and my back yard, but they'd been removed to accommodate more parking. I remembered hitting balls there with Mom, when I was twelve or so. She didn't play well, but she adored Rod Laver. I rubbed my arms. The day was cool for early fall. I think it had rained and yet everything seemed surprisingly arid. "Dust thou art and unto dust thou shalt return." True enough. All cried out, I felt like a piece of fruit made indestructible by some appliance you might buy from the *Home Shopping Network*, use once, then forget about. Apricot jerky, perhaps, or an apple chip. I watched Vicki sob and understood that her emotion was purer than mine. She'd known Mom a brief but intense period of time; she'd had the last measure of Mom, distilled to its essence.

Perhaps this was a cultural problem. I knew from my work that different cultures prepare themselves differently, or not at all. It's complicated. But who doesn't anticipate death in the elderly? Life ends. That's the only thing we can agree on. Certainly knowing that simple fact should help us prepare. It's shocking when it does not.

After a moment, I went to Vicki. My sisters joined me. Because that's how we do things. I placed a hand on her back. She turned and hugged me, hugged each of us. I would never be like Vicki, I thought; I would never have the luxury of such rich clear feeling expressed publicly and precisely. I come from different stock. My sisters and I descend from a long line of women who tough it out, suck it up, and huff ambivalence with every breath. My grandmother taught my mother, her mother taught her, my mother taught me. We are American women, the lot of us, daughters of more than one revolution; we've buried loved ones in these plains since the 1600's. Stoicism comes easily to the ambivalent. My mother's family had been poor and depressingly dour until this past generation. That's when Dad and his cronies arrived, pumped up on ambition fed by the Great War, seeking and finding opportunities and giving us the chance we needed to laugh, at long last. I gazed at the overcast sky that had only begun to break. Faint streaks of blue split the gray, promising something beyond the gloom of the day. It felt like a little gift, a heavenly surprise. *Thank you, Mom.*

My daughters Beatrice and Ruthann put their arms through mine and together we walked to the car. We would have a luncheon for my mother at the club where she'd played golf for over fifty years. Still, I marveled at Vicki's public display. It seemed like performance art: a statement of high anguish. I didn't know what to make of it. Her loss was genuine—she'd cried before, big heaving sobs. But I kept my sobs in. My sisters kept theirs in. Silence best held the grief I understood.

# Two

A flurry of activity followed Mom's death and burial. My sisters and I, along with our adult children, quickly dispensed with her effects. In a matter of days, we divvied up her jewelry, purses, hats, linens, and furniture, keeping most, pitching some, giving much away. We were marvels of efficiency. Mom had liked jewelry, acquiring quite a bit over her ninety-three years. Most was long out of style. What we didn't want we decided to melt down and make into identical bangle bracelets for ourselves, her four daughters; they would bind us together, as if she hadn't already.

And then it was over. Mom died on a Wednesday afternoon, the wake was Friday, the funeral Saturday morning. We cleaned out her condo on Saturday and Sunday. By Tuesday, we were mostly finished. Somehow I had been made executor, perhaps when I wasn't paying attention or because of it. But all of a sudden, the out-of-towners had left town. My sister and brother-in-law drove to Florida. The nieces and nephews returned to their homes out of state. My daughter, Bea, resumed her coursework; Ruthann flew back to Georgia. And Mom was gone for good. I felt suddenly and irrevocably grown up, as if I'd ridden a catapult into adulthood after playing make believe for thirty years. Despite surviving a life-threatening brain aneurysm, a lethal divorce, raising two kids and a daily tread through the mine-field of medicine that I called a career, I had finally—at the age of fifty-two—*matured*. Like many physicians my age and in my line of work, I had a graveyard behind me full of patients who'd died or nearly died while in my care. Esther, Miriam, Nathaniel, Mark, the patients whose names I never knew or couldn't recall, plus dozens, no *hundreds* more—they'd taken their toll but they hadn't done *this*. *This* was something else. The woman who stared back at me in the mirror no longer looked or felt like a kid mistakenly trapped inside an adult's body. I'd become the age on my driver's license. I read somewhere that when both your parents have passed, there's nothing to stand between you and death. But that wasn't it at all. No one had protected me from anything for a long time—I'd been a grown-up since pre-school. This was different. I felt old and looked tired. Was this what it meant to be an orphan? If so, it was awful.

I took to my bed.

I like the way that sounds: *I took to my bed*. It implies that I acted with style and flourish, perhaps adorned with a pink satin bed jacket. It suggests that I knew what I was doing. But I didn't. I only know how to tell the tale.

In the days and nights after my mother died, I spent all my available time in bed. But I couldn't sleep. Mostly, I read. I went back to work after a week, and any time of the day or night I was not working, I slipped under the covers. I forgot to eat. I didn't pay the bills or answer the phone. I managed to walk and feed my dog Olga because she stuck her snout into my ribcage or under my elbow to remind me that she required some upkeep even if I didn't. I read and occasionally drifted off. My choice of material wasn't spiritual, escapist, or inspirational. I didn't read the newspaper or any one of the books that sits in a pile on the unoccupied half of my king-sized bed. I skipped the poetry collections of Collins, Auden, Ryan, and Rilke heaped on my bedside table. I ignored my stash of *New Yorkers*, *Economists*, and *New York Times Sunday Magazines* from weeks past. Nope, I read Harvard Business School case studies. I did homework.

~

I remember my father telling me, on numerous occasions, that the readings at our Catholic Mass were just metaphors I should not take literally. They were just *stories*. "Think of what the story means, in the larger sense. Probably none of these things actually happened."

I come from a family of storytellers.

~

Four months before Mom died I had signed up for an Executive Education course called *Managing Healthcare Delivery* that spanned nine months and required travelling to Boston for three separate weeks. I had enrolled somewhat impulsively near the end of my mother's inexorable decline from dementia, when I could hardly stand the pain of it anymore: her slow disappearance, the wait for her inevitable demise. Every visit to see her grew more challenging. I couldn't bear to be with her; I missed her in her presence. How do you watch someone die backward, regressively, from old age into infancy, without wanting to scream out loud at the injustice? It went on forever and grew worse by the day. Vicki made *pansit*, a traditional Filipino noodle dish, for me most weeks. Comfort food. Sometimes egg rolls too. Mom didn't eat them. The food worked though. It felt like the kindest thing anyone had ever done for me. And when I could not stand my own conflict—my need to fix things and to flee simultaneously—I thought, incongruously, *something is wrong with this picture*. I've spent a lifetime in medicine—*why can't dying be better than this?* And so I looked to Harvard Business School to find the answer. Because—I don't know—where else do you look? The answers were not at the hospital or anywhere in medicine that I could see. I had not found them by going to Mass. I'd searched my soul; it offered no clues.

The Harvard course began one month after Mom's death, which seemed fortuitous but was completely accidental. I'd always been an excellent student so I had to prepare. I did all the required reading in advance. I even bought new highlighters. As part of the preparation, I was required to take the Meyers-Briggs[ii] personality test online. I vaguely remembered the test from when my sister Beth was in graduate school in psychology; she was always referring to me with letters. *I...N...T...J*.

~

"Stories are at the center of culture," Daniel McAdams states in his book *The Redemptive Self: Stories Americans Live By.*[iii] "Stories teach us how to live and what our lives mean. Self and culture come to terms with each other through narrative." In his book, McAdams examines how and why we tell the narratives of our lives in the ways that we do. He looks at highly generative adults who, in middle age, attempt to understand why they've come to be the people they are and why they believe what they believe. He sees the American experience as being individualistic as opposed to other, particularly Eastern, cultures that value collective ethics. He explores the life story, which he refers to as the "narrative self," and analyzes its redemptive nature. The typical American story is that of a special sort of childhood, of some hardship overcome, which leads to a desire to achieve, to help others, and to work hard. The redemptive self is a story that links the individual person to a larger culture: who am I in relation to this society I came from?

~

Lying in bed, I slogged my way through the material for the first of three learning modules, which dealt with the design and leadership of a successful organization. In a month's time I covered over five hundred pages. I learned about the challenges facing the U.S. healthcare delivery system; they seemed *insurmountable.*

I learned about strategy; I learned about cardiac care for the poor in India, cancer care at MD Anderson, orthopedics at Rittenhouse, Duke's heart failure program, Dana-Farber's famous chemotherapy overdose of a Boston Globe reporter, and how to redefine health care in terms of value. I liked that they used the case study method to impart these lessons. Weren't case studies just an elegant form of storytelling?

In the weeks following my mother's death, I was easily distracted and got lost in the details of my reading. I took

Olga for long walks in Lincoln Park then started over, again and again. Some paragraphs I read four, five, even six times. In my grief, I highlighted *everything*. When I arrived in Boston one month later, I realized, to my chagrin, that I had acquired a lot of complex, often contrasting information, but not much sense of the overall picture. I felt muddled by the minutiae.

Stories had always clarified life for me. Narrative gave me the ability to organize my thoughts, to put my principles in order. But my parents' deaths and the uneasiness I felt with my role as a physician had deprived me of my usual facility with narrative. Why, exactly, had I come to Boston? I suppose I wanted the Harvard faculty to weave this story together with the questions I asked myself every day. These were smart people. I felt hopeful it would happen; I would learn something worthwhile. I would learn something that helped make *sense* of the suffering, the waste, the inequity. These disparate worlds—my personal world of micro-managing my mother's death from a silent, ubiquitous killer, my other world of hospital-based healthcare, and the theoretical business philosophy of national healthcare—surely were not as far apart as they seemed. I felt relatively positive that in nine months I would come to understand how they fit together. At the very least, I would learn something of practical value. That's all I wanted.

~

Storytelling turns out to be its own form of redemption, as well as a process of discovery and explanation. We use it to illuminate the zigzag nature of our lives and our loves. Stories evolve over time, from childhood into adulthood and beyond. Each decade we add meaning and every achievement adds purpose. Loss brings perspective of a different sort. And as we age, we think about our legacies. I tell my stories in order to make myself understood and to understand the world around me. Stories seem intrinsic to understanding our heritage; how else do we make sense of history and our place within it? My father believed in the power of metaphor; he told metaphorical stories. My mother's stories were more linear. They both would have agreed with McAdams, however; suffering made them the people they became.

~

"It's not really *the body of Christ*," Dad whispered as we made our way to the Communion rail one Sunday morning during third grade. "It's a wafer. Just think of it as a symbol. Probably made somewhere in New Jersey."

# Three

I've never been to Beijing but they say on bad days the smog can be suffocating, even cause you to lose your bearings. I think of dementia that way, like living in Beijing, not understanding the language or the symbols, where nothing is familiar and the very air you breathe leaves you senseless. During Mom's last few years, I often felt it myself. Overwhelmed I guess. Or in sympathy with her condition.

One day after work I knocked on Mom's door then let myself into the condo with my key. I planned to visit her briefly, then drive downtown for an appointment with my therapist. I needed therapy because I suffered from cognitive dissonance.[iv] Or at least that was the diagnosis I'd given myself. His diagnosis might have been somewhat different.

Perhaps I didn't really need psychotherapy; perhaps I just liked having someone to talk to. Which seemed mostly consistent with a diagnosis of cognitive dissonance. Regardless, my therapist provided a constant, non-crazy person to relate to without having to worry that my problems would upset him. Or if he got upset, it was okay because I paid him. Usually, though, I tried not to upset him.

For the past several years, I had read about *cognitive dispositions to respond* or CDRs, which are forms of bias in medical reasoning and decision-making that can lead to wrong diagnoses. It's a fascinating field of research that seems like it should extend broadly into many disparate areas, well outside of medicine. I knew I'd made some bad decisions over the years even though they seemed responsible, maybe even brilliant at the time. I assumed the same was true not only for other people but for institutions as well. So I'd chosen a bright, highly recommended therapist in the hopes that he might help me sift through my expert rationalizations and move beyond them.

On this visit to my mother's, she sat in her favorite seat

beneath a large picture window, in a blue upholstered chair that rocked ever so slightly, every which way. It was summertime. She had the A/C off and the temperature hovered around seventy-eight degrees. She wore jeans and a flannel shirt. Her gray hair still had a nice wave.

"How you doing, Mom?" I yelled at her.

"Hanging in there," she said with a half-smile. That was her answer to every inquiry about her wellbeing. *Hanging in there.* Usually she prefaced the answer with a long "Ooh," which sounded melodic, resigned, and vaguely upbeat all at once. "And how are you, Margaret?"

"I'm fine." I had to yell, because she couldn't hear much with or without the hearing-aids anymore. But when I heard her say my name I felt that a crisis had been averted, which meant an important piece of her mind remained intact. For the moment, anyway. "I just came from work," I said.

"Oh, you came from work?" Mom's habit of repeating my statement with a question had become increasingly familiar as her mastery of the present diminished. She tried to hide her short-term memory loss. The dementia had occurred over years though it was hard to be exact. Whose memory did that speak to? I thought back and wondered what constituted normal aging and what did not. When had this begun, exactly? Dementia seemed viral, definitely contagious. I forgot things all the time. Could I blame my mother? Sometimes I forgot to take Kleenex and wear sunscreen on my bike rides. I often forgot cilantro for the corn and mango salad I made umpteen times each summer. The signs of dementia are subtle until one knocks you flat. We had just begun having the retirement facility's nurse visit daily to check on Mom. The nurse argued with me about everything. She wanted to lock up Mom's medications in a suitcase. Mom threw a fit when she heard about it. I knew she'd pick the lock. I had to negotiate with both of them. We agreed to a suitcase, but kept it open. Like that made any sense.

I walked over to Mom and kissed her cheek. Age had shrunk

her, bent her spine, thickened her, stiffened her. It had spared her beauty, however. Her skin still felt soft; her face held few lines. I reached over her head and flipped on the air conditioning.

"I did come from work," I said. "What's going on with you?"

"Oh, I'm not feeling too well today, honey." I put a hand to her head and didn't feel a fever. She looked pale but then she hadn't spent time in the sun in over three years.

Not feeling too well could denote any number of things. It usually signaled bowel issues. One of the problems with her memory loss was that she forgot what she should eat, what she shouldn't eat, when she'd eaten, and what hunger or fullness felt like. So dietary indiscretion was the norm. And she refused to wear Depends. Or she didn't remember needing them. She could be surprisingly selective about what she forgot.

"I have to use the bathroom," she said in a rush. She pushed herself out of her chair. I helped her walk there, less than ten steps away. She didn't make it to the toilet.

I suppose the good news is that I eventually arrived at my therapist on time and did not have to think hard to find something to talk about that day. And I can deal with it—the role reversal, I mean. I have cleaned my share of everything, can handle all manner of human fluids and waste. We are simple, common flesh.

The bad news is that after inserting every afflicted item of clothing and bath linen into the washer, I found a sponge and began to bleach the bathroom. I realized that this explosion had precedent. The evidence was old and dried and hard, but present. On the floor and on the walls. In every nook and cranny. I found poop that had splattered above eye level. I'm fairly tall. I tried to remember what principles of physics they'd taught us back in college that might apply. I'd barely passed physics, but still. Perhaps the four laws of thermodynamics pertained; perhaps those were the laws I needed to remember. Could entropy account for this? I found poop that had splashed so hard as to make two, possibly three ninety-degree turns. What were the physics of a splash? I tossed the sponge in favor of a scrub brush. All along I thought I should have paid more attention to electricity, specifically resistors. A little knowledge of electricity seems useful in life—if you want to install dimmer switches, overhead fans, change out light fixtures. You definitely want to know about fuses—I'd learned that one the hard way. But as it turned out I knew even less about physics than I'd ever suspected.

Mom rested in her chair. I felt like a janitor with post-traumatic stress disorder. She told me I was her angel. Did angels have trouble juggling conflicting thoughts and emotions? Did they obsess over the mechanics of their decision-making? I wanted to take a shower and go lie down in a womb somewhere. I wanted never to grow old. I wanted to have someone love me enough to never let it happen. But that someone didn't exist. Not for me, not for her. And I loved her a lot.

She kissed me twice. I hugged her hard and tried not to let her see me cry. She laid her head back and rested again. I thanked God that the memory of it would be gone within minutes. It would have never happened. With someone else to clean for her, the incident would leave her mind sooner than if she'd had to clean up after herself. I thought about my sister Bonnie who frequently took Mom out to restaurants and had similar experiences in public. Bonnie is a better woman than I.

After washing the bathroom and then myself, I made certain that Mom was comfortable and had instructions for her evening meal. I had no doubt she would promptly forget what I told her, so I wrote it down. Usually she found my instructions several days later and called, asking what I had meant by 'Bananas, rice, applesauce, and toast'. I kissed her again and sped downtown to see my therapist. He told me a horror story about his own elderly parents. They had one set of senses between the two of them. He told me he'd planned for his own old age. He'd bought a gun.

"*You bought a gun?!?* Are you kidding me? You're not supposed to tell me that." I was appalled. I counted on him to be the sane one.

He shrugged.

I stared out the floor-to-ceiling windows. I thought about the gunshot wounds I saw in the trauma patients at work; they were usually self-inflicted and often in the elderly. I didn't tell my therapist when it happened because there was no reason to ruin his day too. I thought about Nathaniel, the patient whose dementia and prostate problems had made his daughter nearly insane with anxiety. Maybe dementia is a special kind of disease, a projectile disease, designed to particularly torture the loved ones. Who could think that up? Outside the office window, the setting sun reflected off the buildings along the Chicago River. The light had turned the sky a mystical, otherworldly deep blue, the hypnotizing color of pollution at dusk.

I left the office feeling more relaxed, if not actually better. My therapist was perfect for me. He understood cognitive dissonance because he had it himself. It's the thinking person's alternative to pulling the trigger.

Around this time I turned fifty. As a gift, two friends bought me a session with a famous astrologer. I naturally thought the entire idea was ludicrous. I'd spent my whole career in a scientific field—specifically medicine, sub-specifically anesthesiology—which does not lend itself to astrological interpretation or intervention. That isn't to say those of us in medicine don't acknowledge that more crazy stuff happens when there's a full moon. But I've never been one who "believed" in astrology. I occasionally read my horoscope in the newspaper mostly because it was next to the *Jumble*. It never seemed to reveal anything meaningful. But I was at a low point; dementia takes its toll on family as well as on the afflicted. Besides, I figured the astrologer could make an educated guess as to whether there might be love in my future. I obviously wanted a pass on long life if it involved senility and I didn't much care about fortune, as I knew that work suited me better than leisure. Leisure—in my case—usually meant bug bites, puffy eyes, and large credit card bills. I made particularly bad decisions when idle. I'd read articles about people who won the lottery; it ruined most of them. So I knew better than to relax and let tranquility destroy me. But who didn't want love?

Out of curiosity I visited the astrologer—a doughy woman with thinning hair—who worked in a Chicago office south of the river near the old Carbide & Carbon building. She recorded our conversation and spoke with startling accuracy about my past. She stated that my birth circumstances were unusual and I didn't fit the typical description for my sign. I had been born in the brief time span between a lunar and a solar eclipse. "Your life must seem fated," she murmured, her voice deceptively bland. "As if life pushes you in a particular direction." I had not thought of my life as 'fated' as much as a litany of incredible coincidences. Sometimes I had an uncanny ability to see signs that strangely forecasted events, even warning of imminent danger. I typically ignored them.

"Taurus fits you better," she said. "Read that horoscope in the paper." Perfect. I'd been reading the wrong horoscope my whole life. No wonder it seemed useless.

"There's something highly significant about your chart, an unusual division of the elements. You have four planets in air signs—it gives you an uncanny ability to communicate, and extreme curiosity. You're mentally young for your age. Quality or modes—five are in fixed signs—that's a sign of tenacity, not an Arian quality. The downside of tenacity is that you don't know when to let go. You need to learn to trust your intuition. Even if intuition goes against what you've been told." I agreed with her that I didn't know when to let go. But my intuition was better than I thought? What if my intuition told me not to trust my intuition?

"You have lots of planets in work. Innovation, creativity, research. You like finding things out and putting a different spin on it," she said.

"Between now and April 9, 2013, there's a new development level. Then a static period. Until the new moon in 2016. You'll want to lay the groundwork for any creative work before 2013. There will be a lot of wasted time and energy during those three years. You'll feel guided by others. Use it to do inner work. Maybe go to an ashram. You'll want to have flowers, perhaps buy some property."

I had to ask. "What about love?"

"I don't see much happening with your Venus. Have you tried Internet dating? That might work for you."

I had tried Internet dating. It did not work for me. I was actually writing a book about how it did not work for me, among other things.

One other thing the astrologer mentioned—I should prepare for my mother's demise.

Each time I visited Mom, I stopped at the grocery store first. I would call from the car and she would give me a list of things to buy. Then I went to the Jewel and bought half the things she needed. Later I went back to the store to get the things she'd forgotten. I did this every week not because her memory deteriorated, although it did, but because I kept hoping that the deterioration was temporary. After Vicki moved in, I only had to make one trip because Vicki would give me a complete list. Usually the list included a box of Depends. Only Vicki could get Mom to wear Depends.

I liked going to suburban grocery stores. Or rather I liked going to a single suburban grocery store. In the city of Chicago sales tax is higher, parking is a nightmare, and getting groceries into my building requires more steps than launching the space shuttle. On the other hand, suburban grocery stores tend to grow freakishly large. They carry every food item made except the ones I usually buy in the city. While shopping for my mother I typically spent an hour walking in circles looking for the same items I bought the week before. This was due to an organizational layout that defied comprehension or memorization. A pharmacy had been attached to the grocery store, further confusing the issue, and the products that I used to know where to find in the grocery section ended up being sold in the pharmacy. Like liquor. Why would wine be located in the pharmacy? It's not like it's good for you. Maybe it's because booze makes you feel better in a way similar to calamine lotion or witch hazel. Sympathy cards are placed next to batteries. Think about it.

It did not bother me to buy Depends at the grocery store. I bought them for my aunt when she was alive, then for my mother, and I'm sure I'll buy them for my sisters and for myself when the time comes. They are just large sanitary napkins with bad branding.

One sunny spring day I was in the checkout line with lactose-free milk, a box of Raisin Bran, a loaf of multi-grain bread, some boiled ham, Mom's favorite cheese, and a box of Depends. The adult diapers were the last item to be rung up.

The cashier looked to be about my age. About fifty. We could've easily gone to school together and been part of the same stoner crowd which I'd thankfully survived and left behind. She passed the Depends over the bar code reader, then leaned across the conveyer belt and placed a warm hand gently on my arm. She looked me squarely in the eye. I saw deep compassion in her lined face and not a trace of humor.

"Would you like me to put these in a brown paper bag for you?" she asked, nodding slightly, girl-to-girl, stoner-to-stoner, eyes never leaving mine.

I realized in that split second that she had decided the Depends were for me. They were mine. I was the leaker. I was fifty and leaking; it showed plainly on my face. In that moment, I knew there was nothing I could say or do to convince this woman of my actual continence—she wouldn't believe me anyway—and so I simply showed my appreciation for her empathic treatment of my problem. I nodded. "Thank you," I said. "That would be great." I laughed all the way to the car.

My mom's dementia taught me to open my heart again—nothing breeds humility like helplessness. Her helplessness made me humble. Or maybe it was the other way around. But I learned to let people be nice to me. Even if it means they think I'm incontinent. I'm sure one day I will be. So it helps to laugh about it. In fact, laugh whenever possible. As for the gun issue, I'll get to that later.

For some reason, I returned to the astrologer shortly after my fifty-first birthday. Once again, I heard good things about my career. Always about my career. I heard about making connections, about my healing abilities. When I was born, Saturn was in a good place, career-wise. This would be life-long. The astrologer told me there was nothing happening with my Venus. Like I didn't know that. Nor did she see it happening in the foreseeable future. And this woman looked very far into the future. She mentioned things that were going to happen in 2017. She said there would be unpleasantness around the 23rd of September, 2010. That turned out to be the day after Mom died. Not the 22nd of September. So the astrologer was off by a day. No wonder I never believed in that stuff.

# Four

Mom's condo was part of a retirement community that provided two meals a day, weekly cleaning, and laundry service with the monthly assessment. You could pay extra for certain amenities, like having a nurse stop by once a week, once a day, or multiple times a day and hover—tapping her foot impatiently—while your parent took her medications as slow as humanly possible and with her face set just so. There were additional charges for bathing and hair care. For a fee your mom could take the bus service to the local grocery store as well as a number of different churches and medical centers, wander around, get lost, then get picked up again after having no recollection of where she'd been or what she'd done. The retirement community offered organized activities such as bingo, musical events, movies, and sing-a-longs. Mom didn't participate until her dementia advanced and Vicki encouraged her. Vicki could get her to enjoy herself. I didn't have the patience.

~

When Mom turned ninety my sisters and I took her to Florida to celebrate her birthday. We lost her at a shopping mall in Boca Raton.

It turns out that losing old people is a major problem. Those with dementia have a tendency to wander off, or even drive off. Time is critical and the outcome is often bad, meaning they are found dead. My sister Beth and I sat together in the shoe department at Nordstrom—Beth was trying on something comfortable, expensive, and ugly—when I let Mom walk to the bathroom by herself. Because I didn't have the patience to take her. After all, I could see the entrance to the Ladies Room from my chair; it was less than fifty feet away. And we—I— still managed to lose her. Luckily, we were at an indoor mall, I remembered exactly what she was wearing, and the mall was in

Florida where losing-old-people happens with some frequency. Security uses Segways, allowing them to find missing persons with a reassuring rapidity. They found Mom within twenty minutes—she'd wandered amazingly far in a short period of time—and without her realizing she'd been misplaced. Mom survived my neglect. But what did it mean, cognitively? She took a wrong turn, it could happen to anyone.

~

Over thirty years ago I met a woman who had critical lessons to impart about caring for an elderly parent. If I'd been paying attention, I might have learned them. They were all wrapped up in one brief experience, one night long ago. But I got the lessons wrong. It took years before I understood.

The woman stood silhouetted in the soft light coming from the doorway of her father's hospital room. I was mid-way through my internship year. Though she told me her name, I would forever think of her as the conductor's daughter; I would always remember her as *Nathaniel's daughter*.

It was near midnight and I'd just gotten round to eating dinner: a tuna salad on whole wheat sandwich, the remains of which were room temperature, runny, and stuffed into the back pocket of my scrub pants. Nathaniel's daughter wore elegant clothes, but her suit hung rumpled, as if she'd been caught in the rain then fallen asleep. Dirt streaked her Ferragamos with their iconic buckles and low heels, the rich woman's version of a sensible shoe. She stood still, wraith-like, hands clasped. As I approached, I noted the scent of something herbal. Patchouli? Somewhere I'd read that as few as four molecules of a given substance can be perceived by a sensitive nose. My nose is not only sensitive; I can smell disaster at the molecular level.

~

I don't consider us lucky that Mom wandered off at the mall that afternoon in 2007, but we were fortunate that it happened when my sisters and I were together. We were forced to deal with it. We recognized that Mom had crossed into a territory beyond which there was no turning back. *This was new.* The implications, the inconvenience, and the cost of this next giant step forward seemed enormous. But convincing our mother that she needed a caregiver would require another *two and a half years.* We had to balance her safety against her dignity, her security against her autonomy. Role reversal took on complex layers of meaning. We used the utmost care in how we approached various issues— her medications, her checkbook, her finances—and each of us did it differently with equally poor results. We had already taken away her car after she'd broken her neck while playing golf at the age of eighty-eight. She wanted to maintain what precarious independence she had left. Who could blame her?

~

"*There* you are, Doctor." The Ferragamo woman, older but vulnerable somehow, oddly dispossessed, went from still to a flurry of animated motion, as if life had placed her on pause and my arrival pushed her play button. "Thank God you're here!"

~

Dementia doesn't look the same every day to every person. It doesn't always sound like anything out of the ordinary over the phone. Mom had days when she could carry on a conversation as if she were twenty years younger, days when she remembered the names of all her grandchildren, where I worked, all the details of her past life and mine. And on those days, I agreed with her that she did not need a caregiver. But then she would ask me a question about a topic we had discussed just moments before. Her short-term memory could turn itself off and on and off, unpredictably. The ability to remember what just happened, where you are and were and what was said allows you to function in ways we implicitly take for granted. Our tendency, as offspring, is to use all the available evidence to underestimate how much our parents have declined mentally—it's a well-described cognitive bias called the *valence effect*, or *optimism bias*. It's also known as *wishful thinking*. In the evenings and at night, Mom often hallucinated. When I called in the mornings, she would describe her hallucinations to me. It's hard to pretend everything is okay when your mom describes a midnight visit from a long-dead dentist.

I try now to deconstruct those experiences with my mother. I thought of myself as levelheaded at the time, but in retrospect I wonder. Dementia plays you like a seesaw, only the fulcrum refuses to stay put. As adult "children," we struggle with how to make decisions for the parents who once made decisions for us. We often depend on physicians but aren't certain who to trust because of the conflicting information and advice we're given. The flip side of wishful thinking is to err on the side of caution, which unfortunately means being hamstrung by guilt and doing too much of everything, whether it's indicated or not. Who wants that kind of medical care?

~

The bedraggled woman grabbed my hand and pulled me into the room where an old man lay on a hospital bed. His eyes were closed; his mouth was open. We call this the "O" sign. Commonly seen en route to the "Q" sign.

"My father's miserable." She gestured toward him, still grasping my hand in hers. "I hope you can help him."

"What seems to be the problem?" Looking down at our joined hands, I felt the moist scratch of her freshly bitten cuticles. I used to bite my cuticles, too. Working one week in a hospital cured me forever. "Hello, sir," I said to the patient while disengaging from the daughter.

"His name is Nathaniel," she spoke low and directly into my ear. "Nathaniel Corpisi. You've probably heard of him."

"Hunh," I said.

"He can't urinate."

"Okay. Let me go and grab his chart. I'll be right back."

"But *Doctor*," her jaw clenched tight, "you *are* going to do something, aren't you?" She grabbed me again, both hands on my forearm, twisting. The patchouli, at close range, was potent—way more than four molecules. "You *are* going to help my daddy! He is a very famous conductor, you know. He's conducted some of the finest symphony orchestras in the world, traveled everywhere. We spent holidays in Russia, Vienna, London, and he was the visiting conductor for an entire season in Paris. *I can't stand to see him suffer!*"

~

Early in the summer of 2009, I contacted a man named Robert who had recently started a caregiver agency. My sister Bonnie and I met with him in the lobby of the retirement community where Mom lived.

"Perhaps you could ask your mother to train someone to work with the elderly," Robert suggested as a way to gently deceive Mom into allowing someone to help her. "I ran into the same problem with my mom. She didn't want anyone in her home, even though she clearly needed help."

We took Robert's advice, slowly introducing a young caregiver into our mother's life. Mom wanted none of it. Over a month and with a lot of verbal maneuvering, she gradually, begrudgingly and without her usual grace, came to accept the intruder's presence in her home. We started with four hours a day, five days a week. She fired the woman six times. And then one night in August of 2009, Mom fell out of bed and broke her arm.

The nurse where Mom lived called Bonnie first, and called

the ambulance second. I arrived at the local hospital when they had been in the emergency room for an hour. Dr. Helms, Mom's geriatrician, had decided to admit her because the pain medication made her more confused and ambulation would be an issue. She had broken her proximal humerus, just below the shoulder, which meant she could not push herself out of a chair. Luckily, she didn't require surgery.

~

I moved to the far side of the Nathaniel's bed and smiled down at him. It was an automatic smile, a middle-of-the-night, neural reflex smile, disconnected from the muscles of empathy. The conductor did not respond.

I felt his belly, a massively distended bladder, and got a good whiff. Dueling molecules. I turned to the daughter.

"He'll probably need a catheter placed."

"Won't that be painful?" Her eyelid twitched rhythmically.

"He'll feel *much better* once his bladder's emptied," I said more gently. I made a conscious effort to slow down, to interrupt the momentum that carried me through these call nights and safeguarded precious sleep. "I'll be right back." I also needed to finish the tuna sandwich before my stomach ate itself.

"But wait!" She moved to the bedside. "Let me show you something!"

She yanked her dad's blanket down, pulled back his hospital gown. Then, reaching into his crotch, she grabbed his shriveled penis and pulled it straight up, like a fisherman showing off a prize catch.

"You see?" She pointed to the skinny, elongated wiener stretched taut in her hand. I nodded. "I think he's got a dorsal vein thrombosis!" she said, eyes filling. "Wouldn't that explain it? His symptoms? I think that's what it is! A dorsal vein thrombosis. I've read about it. See how his penis is purple? See how that purple thing goes up and down there?"

I nodded. I'd never heard of a dorsal vein thrombosis. Even with his dick in the air, the old man didn't flinch. I stood bobbing my head like a dog on a dashboard.

I felt tired, old and young, brittle and limp. Not cut out for this line of work. The smells. The sadness. I didn't have a mom or a dad or any relatives who were doctors; I didn't inherit the trade secrets. I dropped into the chair behind me, and then remembered the tuna.

I stood and felt for my back pocket. Tuna salad juice had seeped through my pants and underwear.

"Why don't you go ahead and put that down now," I heard myself say, distantly, the words slow and elongated inside my ears. I gave my head a hard shake and waved vaguely at the old man's baton. "I'm going to call the urology resident, 'cause, uh, he has more experience than I do with this sort of thing." A stream of tuna juice crept slowly down my leg until it reached the top of my right knee sock.

~

Mom, Bonnie and I waited hours in the ER before we were taken to Mom's hospital room. They had assigned her to a general medicine/oncology floor. Because of her age and dementia, she was given a room near the nursing station. Bonnie and I had warned the nursing staff that she might wander, was at high risk for falling, and was likely to become increasingly confused by the unfamiliar environment. A number of nurses and aides came and went, trying to get her settled as the afternoon shift change approached.

I asked a nurse if we could bring up the guardrails on the bed so that Mom would not fall out.

"No, we don't elevate guardrails on beds anymore. That's considered a violation of patients' rights. We have an alarm system that we put in place if you think she is likely to get out of bed."

"What kind of alarm system?" I asked.

"There's a sensor on the bed," the woman pointed to a pad under the sheet. "We just hook that up. And then we place a pad on the floor beside the bed. We'll push the bed itself next to the wall so that she can't get out that way. The pad senses when she moves off of the mattress, and the pad on the floor has a sensing system also. It's illegal to 'confine' patients now."

I tried to take this in. Make sense of it. "So basically Mom is free to fall out of bed, get injured, and then the alarm will sound. But she would be illegally confined if we put up the side rails to prevent her from falling out in the first place. She has the right to be harmed, but not be confined," I said.

There is no way that one system fits all patients, neither in concept nor in implementation. To protect some, we harm others. The rights of patients, as defined by politicians, were a rabbit hole.

"Well, no... the alarm sounds when she starts to leave the bed and someone at the nurses' station hears the alarm and comes into the room," the nurse assured me.

Maybe I look stupid. I don't think I look stupid, but I'm often underestimated. I think it's the blond hair. But I'm much smarter than I look. And I'd spent decades in hospitals listening to alarms go unattended at empty nursing stations. Hospitals—*nationwide*—have staffing issues. Let's not pretend here. I don't know a single person who has ever worked in a hospital who has not had the experience of listening to alarms and call buttons ring and ring and ring. So I knew exactly what this whole scenario meant for my mother. We had a barn door and horse situation. Mom was already disoriented. Hell, I was disoriented! Add some pain medicine and she'd be hallucinating in no time. I closed my eyes and shook my head.

"It's *against the law* to confine someone." I heard stridency in her let-me-tell-you-the-rules voice, the certainty that creeps because if something is illegal, someone somewhere must have given it some thought, right? Instead of what really happens, instead of the massive bureaucratic compromises that actually occur in public policy everywhere particularly as applied to health care. That's how our system works. Never assume common sense has been applied at any step along the way. *Ever.*

"But it's not against the law to prevent them from falling out of bed," I said. I wasn't going to point out the obvious: that was how she'd broken her arm in the first place. And now we had a state law designed to *protect* patients that effectively accomplished the opposite. Doesn't that define the law of unintended consequences?

"We'll keep a close eye on her," the nurse told me.

Right. I knew how that would go. Bonnie or I would need to be there twenty-four hours a day. Or we would have to hire someone. The good news was that Mom's arm hurt enough that she wouldn't use it to try to move around too much right at this moment.

"Can I go through her medications with you? I want to make certain that I have all the orders from Dr. Helms."

I sat down and gave her the list of medications, allergies, food preferences, and then I told her to make certain the chart shows that she is *Do Not Resuscitate.*

The nurse gave me a cold look. "Are you the power of attorney?"

"Yes, I am," I said mildly.

"And I suppose you have the paperwork with you? Is it something you carry in your purse just in case?"

I took a very slow deep breath. I took a cleansing breath. A do-not-lose-your-temper-now or you'll-regret-it and your-mom-will-suffer breath. I searched my heart for my hard-earned clarity with regard to this bullshit. *Where the hell was it?*

"No," I said, "but I can have it faxed if you give me the number. Or I can bring it tomorrow."

"Fine," she said. She spun on her heel and was gone from the room.

This had turned into a completely ridiculous situation. And

I'd made an enemy. My sisters and I decided that we did not want our mother resuscitated in the event of a cardiac arrest. We had discussed it with her physician. He agreed with us.

~

Brisk footsteps announced the midnight arrival of the urology resident, a clean-cut, wholesome, Navy fighter pilot of a doctor. He was a couple years older than I, tougher, wiser, a conservator of charm. He introduced himself to the obtunded conductor and his daughter, then set up the catheter insertion set. He felt Nathaniel's enormous bladder. He went about the urology business without delay, not engaging the daughter who seemed mesmerized by the practiced economy of his actions. He struggled to feed the yellow rubber catheter into the old man's member, past the hypertrophied prostate and into the distended bladder. Finally, with this latest insult, Nathaniel stirred, and a moan of pain escaped him. The daughter dropped to her knees beside the bed, clinging to her father's hand. Tears fell to the front of her blouse. Shudders reverberated through her body; her sobs shook the side rails of the hospital bed, perhaps the hospital itself. Her anguish seemed nothing less than razor-sharp, astonishing. Standing behind her, I shut my eyes against her pain; it reached me anyway. When I looked up, everything had changed: Nathaniel, gorked and up to his eyeballs in piss, appeared to be the lucky one. Not long for this world, a simple rubber catheter would cure his ills. The urology resident would move on to the next enlarged prostate. I would change out of my tuna-scented attire and go home to my family. But Nathaniel's daughter might not recover so quickly.

~

My mother's life, at ninety-two, consisted of spending all day every day in a chair, staring at a television screen, unable to hear the dialogue, unable to read the words that ran across the bottom for the hearing-impaired. She looked forward to visits from family members, and then promptly forgot who visited as soon as we were out the door and complained that no one visited her. She was plagued by arthritis, confusion, loss of memory, and disorientation. Her bowels were completely unpredictable and a source of ongoing embarrassment and distress and pain to her. Until she forgot them too. That pretty much described a typical day. To make matters worse, she knew she was losing her mind and it tortured her. *Imagine what that's like*, she often said.

If she were to have a cardiac arrest, a code blue team would rush into her room, pump on her chest, deliver an electric shock that jolted her entire body, put a tube down her throat, give drugs such as epinephrine, vasopressin, amiodarone, etc. Unfortunately, the rate of successful resuscitation of in-hospital patients over the age of 70 is around12%, though the data are all over the place. Resuscitation is one thing. Survival to discharge is quite another. Data for patients over ninety remain sparse, but are probably in the range of 3-5% survival. That's how many survive the arrest. Very few actually leave the hospital. No one has looked at one- or three- or six-month survival, as far as I know. And I've searched. With a diagnosis of cancer the resuscitation rate is incredibly low, typically less than 5%. The numbers that are available do not parse out the quality of the resuscitation, meaning whether individuals who have been resuscitated are cognitively impaired, or even alert, or back to normal. It is generally assumed that resuscitation means they are simply alive. Our mother's dementia had significantly worsened over the previous four years. Performing cardio-pulmonary resuscitation—it seems safe to assume—would not improve her mental status. If anything, were she to be successfully resuscitated, she would be even less with it than before. And a thirty-year old nurse was trying to shame me for not wanting that type of care for my beloved mother, who already was suffering. I would tell the nurse to go f**k herself, or better yet, educate herself, except that she'd probably take it out on my mom. And the problem really wasn't this one nurse, it was the system that led her to believe that indiscriminate resuscitation constituted appropriate care in the first place.

We live in a society where we act first and think later, or don't think at all, particularly with regard to resuscitation. Everybody gets resuscitated unless it is practically tattooed on your forehead, big oranges signs everywhere, your attorney and your physician at your bedside with legal documents in their hands at the time of your demise to prevent someone from instituting CPR. You could have every single organ system in total shutdown mode and they would still pump on your chest if you hadn't dated the paperwork properly. And resuscitation doesn't even work that well in the vast majority of people.[v]

This is only one example, but it turns out to be an incredibly important example, of how far off-track American healthcare has gone. And I know. I'm part of it. I go to arrests all the time. Our emergency rooms and ICU's are choked with elderly dying patients, often unaccompanied by relatives or paperwork, and nobody knows what to do so everything gets done until a day or two or three later when someone finally reaches a family member who says: *Oh, Mom (or Dad or Auntie or Whomever) didn't want to be resuscitated. We'd talked about it, we just never got around to filling out the paperwork. Please withdraw support!* Resuscitation—by law—is a given; you must actively and with great difficulty opt out. In some states it's nearly impossible. But more importantly, it is not one procedure, but a pathway. It is a pathway that starts simple but grows more complex, and that works well only in particular patients, costs money, often does harm, and—in the best circumstances, meaning in-hospital arrests with high quality CPR and ACLS (Advanced Cardiac Life Support)—results in thirty percent resuscitation. That sounds pretty good, but in fact only about five percent of survivors actually leave the hospital. And those tend to be the people you don't expect to arrest; they usually have something treatable. Published statistics sound better than that, but I don't believe them because I've seen how studies can skew results and it's well documented that people don't want to publish poor outcomes. Don't even get me started on the research paid for by drug companies. There is high variability between studies; in other words, they aren't reproducible. People arrest for a reason.

~

I stepped forward, placed an arm around the disheveled daughter's shoulders and pulled her—not gently—back from her dad, his hospital bed, through the door, and into the hallway. The conductor had ceded control of his orchestra.

"I didn't get your name." I took Kleenex from a pocket and handed it to her. "Let's go for a walk until the catheter's in and your dad is feeling better."

"Thank you, doctor. My name is Anita. Thank you so much for your help."

~

A few days after breaking her arm, Mom left the hospital for the nursing home facility affiliated with and located next door to her retirement community. This nursing home had the same type of alarm system as there had been at the hospital, with the sensor pads on the bed and on the floor. Mom was at the nursing home for no more than a half hour before she fell out of bed and landed on the floor in an attempt to go to the bathroom alone. Because of her dementia, she did not remember to press the call button for assistance. And because of the type of nursing home that it was—average, no better or worse than most—no one would have come anyway.

I called Robert and asked if he had someone available who could care for her twenty-four hours a day. He said yes, and she could begin that evening. Bonnie and I packed Mom up and took her home. From then on, Mom accepted a caregiver without question. That's when Vicki entered our lives. Vicki moved in, giving Bonnie and me a much-needed respite. Mom stopped fighting her battle for independence when Vicki arrived. She became docile. I breathed a sigh of relief at the same time my heart broke and I realized that the astrologer had been correct. The end was coming. Vicki took meticulous, loving care of Mom and Mom instantly adored Vicki. We were lucky that my father had planned ahead and saved enough for his and my mother's old age so that we could afford to pay out of pocket for Vicki. We were lucky in an untold number of ways. It took me a long time to sort through them all.

# Five

Errol Morris, writer and filmmaker, wrote a five-part series on the *New York Times* Opinionator blog in 2010 called "The Anosognosic's Dilemma: Something's Wrong but You'll Never Know What It Is." Morris had interviewed a Cornell professor of social psychology named David Dunning who described a cognitive bias known as the *Dunning-Kruger* effect. To put it bluntly, it states that the incompetent are too incompetent to know how incompetent they are.[vi]

While reading the "Offbeat News" section of the 1996 *World Almanac*, Dunning had found the story of McArthur Wheeler, a bank robber who brazenly walked into banks, held them up, and walked out. He wore no disguise; he simply smiled into the security cameras. As it turned out, McArthur Wheeler had sprayed himself with *lemon juice*, which he believed would render him invisible. He had previously verified the effectiveness of the lemon juice treatment; he'd taken a Polaroid photo of himself after testing the lemon spray and it failed to show an image. Believing he was, in fact, invisible due to lemon juice, this five foot six inch, two hundred seventy pound man proceeded to rob two banks and was immediately apprehended. Lemon juice had not made him invisible *to the police*. Inspired by the story, Dunning designed a study to show that incompetence prevents us from recognizing our incompetence. He named his theory the *Dunning-Kruger* effect.

I love this story, not because it deals with incompetence, but because it proves that people have the power to convince themselves of almost anything. While incompetence is tragic, it is no more tragic than ignorance or denial. Every day, people of all levels of intelligence behave in ways that are ruinous to their health and wellbeing, physically and emotionally. And it isn't as if they don't know better. They usually do. But when they look in the mirror, they are awed by the power of the lemon juice.

Later in the article, Dunning remarks on those amazing words uttered by Donald Rumsfeld: "There are known knowns. These are things we know that we know. There are known unknowns. That is to say, there are things that we know we don't know. But there are also unknown unknowns. There are things we don't know we don't know." Dunning states, "That's the smartest and most modest thing I've heard in a year." Though Rumsfeld specifically referred to terrorism, he might just as easily have been talking about medical care, medical research, the business of healthcare, healthcare reform, behavioral economics, or any of the fields that abut caring for our sick and *healthy* and the massive economic machine that entails. It's hard to search for unknown unknowns because it feels akin to an admission of incompetency or inadequacy; as a result, it becomes a problem for intelligent people in all fields and at all levels of experience. The capable are just as at risk as the incompetent; they assume that intelligence or ability in one field naturally extends to other areas as well. They don't know what they don't know.

I arrived in Cambridge, Massachusetts on Sunday, October 24th, 2010. Although the day was rainy, the colors of autumn would brighten in the week to come. A porter showed me to tiny quarters in the Executive Education housing building, which overlooked the Charles River. We had been divided into study groups prior to our arrival and assigned rooms accordingly. Each study group would occupy a section of housing organized around a central meeting room with a large table, a refrigerator stocked with water and soda, AV equipment, and many electrical outlets. Hallways extended in finger-like projections off the meeting rooms. My dorm room felt chilly and damp until I realized the heater had been disconnected. I removed the control panel and turned on the main switch to get some warmth going. Then I unpacked my clothes, hung everything up, and sat on the bed.

I thought of all the reading I had done to prepare for this course, the overwhelming evidence detailing the countless difficulties underlying an industry that represented seventeen percent of the United States' gross domestic product. I thought of all the reading I had done prior to the course, in healthcare journals, in the business section of the daily paper, in articles about economics for the past two decades. Everyone seems to agree that we have troubles. But when that much money is involved, the way of thinking about problems and solutions gets constricted by the so-called politico-industrial complex. We know we want to fix the system but we don't really want to change it all that much, especially not *our part*, not the part that makes us money. We're all guilty. We want to tweak a monster just a smidge, put up a bumbershoot in a hurricane, then expect miraculous change to occur, like everything will suddenly become affordable. We don't want it to hurt too much. So what can you do in this situation, when it seems as if everyone is wearing the lemon juice?

I guess you go to business school.

~

The first time I stuck a needle in Miriam Lewitsky, I thought she seemed ancient. She had a puffy face, straw-like hair, and bruised, fragile skin. Long-term steroids had caused those changes.

Mrs. Lewitsky was every intern's nightmare—chronically ill, suffering, and, worst of all, the wife of a board member and therefore a VIP.

She'd been admitted three weeks earlier. Her medical attending was Dr. Cruzario, a highly regarded pulmonologist, her husband a weird but wealthy financier. She carried a diagnosis of idiopathic pulmonary fibrosis.

Rona, the resident, had told me on morning rounds to draw an arterial blood gas from Mrs. Lewitsky. So I gathered up the necessary equipment and headed in to meet her.

"Who are you?" she wheezed from dried, purplish lips. Her nasal oxygen cannula sat high on her forehead, sending oxygen to her hairline.

I introduced myself.

"Hullo then, young doctor." She closed her eyes and lay her head back against the pillow. "Fix the pillows for me, would ya?"

I came around to the far side of the bed. She couldn't lean forward on her own; I had to hold her shoulder forward with my right arm while fluffing and repositioning the pillow with my left. She wasn't as light as she looked.

"It's gotta be higher. I don't like it so low."

I pushed her forward again. The hospital gown stuck to her spine and I felt her damp skin through the thin cotton. The back of her stylish red hair was flat from the combination of lying too long in one position, infrequent washing, and accumulated hairspray.

"I suppose you're gonna stick me for something," she rasped. I lowered her back. She hadn't done any work but seemed more out of breath. I put the nasal oxygen back in her nose.

"Well, actually, yes I am. We need to check a blood gas." After nine months of internship, I'd learned to invoke the royal *we* whenever possible. I had no authority and little experience. Calling myself *we* was a semantic attempt at validation, and a surprisingly effective one.

"Don't bother with my right wrist. It's still sore from the last one."

I turned her left hand over and examined the inside of the wrist. Bruises ran halfway to her elbow. I felt for the radial pulse and she flinched.

"It's so sore," she said.

"This is the good arm?" I asked, not feeling any pulse whatsoever.

"The other one's worse."

"There's not much here," I said. "I'm going to take a feel of the other arm. I'll make sure to give you some local."

"A lot of good that does," she said. She was right. The local anesthesia stung and may not have helped, but it made me feel

41

better.

Her right wrist had a weak but detectable pulse. I set up my equipment and prepped her skin.

"Talk to me."

"I beg your pardon?" I said.

"Say something. Tell me a story. I hate this."

Mrs. Lewitsky's eyes were still shut, but sweat broke out on her upper lip. She seemed to be breathing harder, and I could hear an audible wheeze. Her lips looked bluer than before. I hadn't even given her the local yet.

"I get nervous," she said.

"Did I tell you I have a new baby, Mrs. Lewitsky?"

She shook her head slightly.

"Her name is Bea, and she's eleven months old. Her father and I are both blond, but she's a redhead, like you. Can you imagine? From the moment she was born, her hair was bright red. I figured it was the blood, you know? That it would wash off. But it was just herself. I had no idea where a child of mine would get red hair, but my mom says there was lots of red hair in her family, and there's some in my husband's family too, so go figure. My entire pregnancy I was absolutely certain I'd have a blond little girl, but then she came out a redhead. Anyway, now my life is totally dependent on a nanny. Her name is Monica and she's twenty-four..." I kept up the chatter but it wasn't easy. I had to stick her three times before I finally found the artery, small and traumatized from repeated punctures. By the time I finished, Mrs. Lewitsky and I were both covered in sweat, and she'd acquired a detailed account of my life's history. She stayed with me, though. She asked questions and she didn't complain.

"Thanks, honey," she said when I placed the bandage on her wrist.

I didn't know what to say. I nodded and left the room.

~

In Cambridge, Dr. Richard Bohmer introduced himself to the room full of Executive Education enrollees. A balding, thin man, perpetually moving, he had developed the course that would get us thinking about some of the problems that plagued healthcare in America and the ways they might be tackled, if not solved. He originated from New Zealand where he'd earned an MD from Auckland University, then obtained a Master's in Public Health from Harvard. Prior to joining the Harvard Business School faculty over a decade earlier, he'd managed a hospital in the Sudan and run the Quality Improvement program at Massachusetts General Hospital, among other things. This guy had it all—he was an academic with street cred. As part of his work at the business school, he'd literally seen and studied healthcare around the world.

We gathered in the Executive Education building on the Sunday afternoon of our arrival where we'd been assigned seats in a tiered, C-shaped modern classroom that had all the bells and whistles. Reading materials, notepads, and ballpoint pens *that doubled as highlighters* had been placed at each person's place along with a large sign designating our names. Attendees came from parts of Europe, Britain, Africa, India, Australia, South America, Central America, Canada, Singapore, Malaysia, and beyond. Most participants were with groups from their hospitals, either administrators and/or physicians. A few, like me, had come alone. As we entered the room, we wandered about, looking for the seats that had been pre-assigned to us. I found mine in the second row on the left hand side. The names were not in alphabetical order; it did not appear that any rhyme or reason had determined our seating arrangement.

The introductory lecture was delivered in what I would come to appreciate as classic Bohmer style: incisive, enthusiastic, and thought-provoking. He supplied us with insights and then questions about how healthcare currently was being organized, delivered and paid for. He compared healthcare in the U.S. to other first world countries. He provided hard data to show that it did not compare favorably. His intent was for us to apply those questions to our own hospitals, our markets, and make us consider the country as a whole. This was the autumn of 2010. He raised questions without getting political, though the Affordable Care Act was being debated in Congress at the time and we were in Massachusetts, where the template for that legislation had originated. He managed to make his presentations both energizing and incredibly depressing. The problems facing the nation seemed insuperable, both from an economic and a public health perspective. And yet the need to fix the system had never been more urgent. Bohmer used his intricate knowledge of the Harvard affiliated hospitals to serve as a microcosm for healthcare across the country, though in all fairness it is perhaps a small scale version of the best healthcare available in the U.S., where medical malpractice rates are controlled, where the worst healthcare is still better than average, and where the hospitals may cooperate to an extent not seen elsewhere. In a few isolated parts of the country, replication of services has been prevented at tremendous cost savings. Where do these magical places exist outside of Boston? Perhaps only in isolated areas where other large systems prevail, places like the Mayo Clinic, Geisinger, Virginia Mason, Intermountain, and a few others. We would study these systems and learn from them.

Later, I wandered into the welcome cocktail reception and dinner. I slid into an empty seat and made conversation. I'm not good at the meet-and-greet. But the hospital where I work, which did not send me to this course, belongs to a large and well-known healthcare system in Chicago. So people asked me about the implementation of the system's innovative physician group. We were still in the early stages. It had only begun to affect our practice and it was painful, at best. Could I say that? The program had been designed for primary care physicians but was being applied broadly to the specialists as well. I didn't see the big picture yet; it would take some time. It would require my sitting through this very course, actually, before I came to appreciate the prescient changes being made by the very system in which I worked. I thought about what my mother had always said. *If something doesn't make any sense, it's usually about money.* Here was a case in point. But homespun aphorisms at Harvard? I should probably keep my mouth shut. On the other hand, why would I start now?

~

In idiopathic pulmonary fibrosis, a normal lung is gradually replaced by scar tissue. The lungs lose their elastic properties, and breathing gets more and more difficult. There's no known cause and no good treatment. Back then we didn't do lung transplants, at least not often and less often successfully. Mrs. Lewitsky had had an open lung biopsy the year before to verify the diagnosis. She had seen specialists from all over the city. But since no one could figure out the cause, her treatment was nonspecific. She was given corticosteroids in the hope of slowing down the fibrotic process, antibiotics when she was febrile, diuretics when she seemed fluid overloaded, oxygen— what we call, inadequately, supportive care. Unfortunately, the supportive care had side effects. From long-term corticosteroid use, she developed widespread osteoporosis, diabetes-requiring insulin, hypertension-requiring medication. And throughout this period of time, her lung disease didn't improve, or even stay the same. It got worse.

~

Monday morning's lectures covered strategy, both the articulation and implementation thereof. The need to have a business strategy seems obvious, but often gets lost in the details. *What is strategy in healthcare?* It seemed as though there were many levels to strategy, many points of view. *It isn't a typical business,* I mused. *Illness fundamentally interferes with a person's ability to make choices. Wellness, on the other hand, should not. But the economics of life restrict our healthcare choices, just as they do with regard to everything else. The sicker we are, the fewer options we will have. People tend to trust their doctors. Most doctors are trustworthy, but certainly not all. Are insurance companies trustworthy? Are hospitals? Are hospital systems trustworthy? What does that really mean? Who can you count on to put your best interest first, to put your interest in front of their shareholders' or business interest? Isn't that usually an inherent conflict of interest? And—if you could make an informed choice—would you necessarily agree with the way those priorities are ranked? Hospitals and systems routinely fail patients with poor coordination of care. Even the best hospitals with the best doctors often fall into this category. But I was thinking like an educated consumer, an industry insider, not like a provider. I had to think like all three.* Some lectures centered on value as a fundamental healthcare strategy. But value alone doesn't support an unsustainable system. Many lectures dealt with leadership. Several of the leaders presented were essentially turnaround experts; others were visionaries. And healthcare had systems issues and personnel issues just like other industries. Unfortunately, a couple of the impressive leaders we learned about subsequently had been fired or were in prison. That was discouraging.

During the afternoon, we received the results of our Meyers-Briggs personality tests to peruse. Mine sat on the desk in front of me, ticking quietly like an unexploded bomb. I flipped through the pages and saw some nice diagrams, which neatly mapped and dissected my meager social skills. Dr. Jim Dowd gave a lively talk about the nature of personality and how it impacted performance in the workplace. The Meyers-Briggs designation is a series of four letters or preferences, the first of which refers to Introversion and Extroversion. I knew I was an introvert, but it turned out we'd been seated according to personality types. So I sat surrounded by introverts! This explained why we were having so much fun. Dr. Dowd took the time to clarify that an introvert is someone who draws energy from being alone, while an extrovert draws energy from other people. It's a matter of how you recharge your emotional batteries. Then Dr. Dowd, a self-described introvert, asked the group of extroverts if they went out to party after a long, exhausting day, and they all *burst out laughing* in acknowledgment! My seatmates and I were understandably horrified. The second letter in the classification refers to (S)ensing and I(N)tuition, or whether you like information in detailed packages or prefer to interpret and add meaning. I scored high in the Intuition category, meaning I like to take information in, mull it over, and think about the broader applications. I remembered the astrologer telling me the same thing. The third preference is (T)hinking and (F)eeling, which indicates whether you tend to look at a topic with logic and consistency or to focus on the people and special circumstances. I scored high as a thinker. This did not surprise me; feelers make me crazy. Again, the astrologer had made the same point. The similarities between the two assessments were startling. And the final preference, (J)udging and (P)erceiving, refers to one's way of relating to the world. I knew I was a *J*; I am a pretty decisive person. I wondered how it could be that astrology and a widely utilized psychological assessment tool based on the principles of Carl Jung would have so much in common. Might there be symmetry in the universe?

At the end of the lecture, Dowd assigned an exercise to help highlight the particular tendencies of the Meyers-Briggs personality types, pitting the detailed-oriented against us big-picture folks. We were divided into small groups. Our assignment: design a party boat for the business school on the Charles River. My group created a glass-bottom gin palace—low slung to slide under the bridges, yet long and elegant enough to handle catering and a live band with a dance floor. Think of a barge on the Seine, slightly smaller, more modern, fueled by hedge-fund money. We had big-time fund-raising in mind, with celebrity charmers like Larry Summers and Bill Clinton on board for the inaugural voyage. Bono would sing, naturally. We didn't bother with the tedious details, we left those up to the *Sensors*, who provided precise measurements, cost estimates, timeframes and so on. Everybody had a great time and the exercise broke the ice among the participants. Afterwards, I glanced through the many-paged discussion of my own test results, and realized that I was a big picture type doing a detail-person's job. Decades ago, I'd chosen the *wrong field* for my personality. No wonder I felt so tired.

~

During the second week of my month with Mrs. Lewitsky, I overheard the resident on the pulmonary service—a bespectacled ass-kisser named Harold—say something about her going home. I didn't understand how this was going to happen, since she seemed more short of breath than ever, but I'd come to recognize that a strange aura surrounded her care. We were actively discouraged from discussing the obvious. Though I was the intern on her case and had the most contact with her, I was often the last to know what was happening.

After two weeks with Miriam Lewitsky, I realized I'd never seen a family member visit. Not even her husband. Then late one night on call, I spotted him sitting at the nursing station. Mr. Lewitsky was a short, pale man with red ears and large psoriatic hands. He sat alone, reading his wife's chart. I asked to speak with him. Then I turned around to answer a page, and, moments later when I turned back, he'd disappeared. It seemed odd that he visited his wife at midnight, when certainly she was asleep and he couldn't expect to find any doctors on the ward. This wasn't a normal family. Normal, I hypothesized, was like the inverse of pornography; I couldn't define it, but I knew what it wasn't.

~

Throughout the week in Cambridge, I listened to each and every lecture closely, though I filtered them through the perspective of my mother's recent death and the care of the elderly as I saw it happening day after day. I thought of the unnecessary suffering—the procedures, the tests, the feeding tubes, the tracheostomies, dialysis being performed on ninety-year-old people with dementia. How often did we see families unable or unwilling to let parents or spouses die? We saw it all the time, the unwillingness to make a person at the end-of-life—someone who is expected to die—*DNR*. It wasn't just the families who thought medicine was capable of offering more than it actually could, it was the doctors who disingenuously promoted the hope that maybe your fragile, elderly loved one could pull off some superhero stunt and regain his previous mental and physical capacities, despite months or even years of obvious decline. It often seemed that the worse or more distant the relationships, the more kneejerk care the patients were given. I was not the only one who felt that way; the sentiment was common among the orderlies and nursing care technicians and nurses all the way to the physicians. And then I listened to the numbers. The last six months of life accounted for roughly twenty-five percent of our Medicare spending[vii]. That is a very important and disturbing statistic. And the number has not gone below twenty-five percent for years. We try really hard to revive the people least likely to benefit.

If resources were unlimited, that might make sense. We have been spending as though we are a country of drunken sailors on leave. But I think we can all now agree, our resources are not unlimited. I no longer believe that obvious questions are obvious to everyone. So I state them plainly: do we want to prolong the painful process of dying? Is that where we want to put our health care dollars?

~

The third week I took care of Mrs. Lewitsky, she began

complaining of back pain. Studies were done to document the spinal compression fractures, which undoubtedly caused her discomfort. I discussed her pain management with Rona, and together we decided to give her oral narcotics, Tylenol #3's. Now when the pulmonary service made rounds with Dr. Cruzario, he spoke less about her care, her diagnosis, new medications, or the odds of getting her home. He seemed less interested in her altogether; perhaps he saw the progression of her disease as a failure. He acted dismissive; he couldn't cure her or even help her so she was no longer a "fascinoma" as we called the curious cases that defied simple diagnosis and treatment. He spoke frequently of the effects the steroids were having on her psyche: crazy, he called her, but I didn't think she was crazy. I thought he was a jerk and she just didn't like him. She didn't hide it because she didn't have to.

A week later, the nursing supervisor informed me she'd scheduled a patient care conference so that everyone involved in Mrs. Lewitsky's care could get together to discuss what to do next. Because nobody knew what to do. She was in a long, slow, untreatable decline: too young to let die, too sick to send home.

Before the conference, I went into her room. Her eyes were closed and her red hair had grown out, showing gray roots. She held her nasal oxygen cannula in her right hand, and the TV remote in her left.

I pulled a chair to the side of the bed and sat down.

I asked how she felt.

She opened her eyes and looked sideways at me without moving her head. "How do you think I feel?"

"How's the pain medicine holding you?" I asked.

"Sometimes it's okay, sometimes I think I need something stronger."

"We can take care of that," I said. I took her hand and turned it over to look at her battered wrist.

"Would you like to go home?" I asked. "Be with your family?"

She met my eyes directly, no longer distant, or reserved, or cold, or preoccupied, or "out of it". She wasn't any of those things I'd thought. She looked unbearably sad. "The kids are away at school. Arnie's at work all the time." She squeezed my hand in hers. "I think I'm better off where I am." I knew then what had eluded me for weeks: Miriam Lewitsky was simply alone. She was completely alone and she was dying. Now I knew. She, of course, had known this all along.

"Okay," I said. "I've got your patient care conference now. Anything you want me to tell them?"

"Nah," she said. "Nothing at all."

I took the nasal oxygen from her hand and hooked it around her ears, positioning the openings inside her nose. The tops of her ears had been rubbed raw from weeks of wearing the cannula.

People in lab coats filled the small conference room. Three nurses, including the head nurse, someone from Utilization Review, a woman from Social Work, her attending pulmonologist, Rona, Harold, and I sat in a rough circle. The meeting began as soon as her doctor sat down.

We discussed Mrs. Lewitsky's course, her lab findings and test results, her current medications and therapies, her prognosis and treatment plan. No one seemed too sure what we should do with her, where she should go. Dr. Cruzario expressed his concern that she was taking too much pain medicine.

"We don't want to make an addict out of her, that would be terrible!" he boomed. Her doctor was short, with pronounced jowls and a history of being listened to.

I waited for Rona to speak up. But she nodded her head at me instead. "But Dr. Cruzario, she isn't getting adequate pain relief with her current regimen," I said. "Her back pain is severe, and the Tylenol # 3 isn't holding her."

He turned in his chair to face me fully. "Young lady," he began. I realized I'd been set up. "This woman has been my patient for several years. She is highly manipulative, crazy from all the steroids, and I know what's best for her. Let's get her off all narcotics, and let's do it soon."

He stood then, looked around once more, which I guessed meant the meeting was over, then started toward the door. But before reaching the door, he stopped in front of where I sat, put one hand on his hip, pointed the other at me, and said in a loud, reproachful voice I will never forget, "Above all, DO NO HARM!"

My first thought, and I think I'm pretty clear on this, was *What a jackass*. My second thought was the recognition that we'd done her plenty of harm already, but we still had a responsibility to relieve her pain. Much of that pain was a direct result of the steroids she'd been given.

I finished my month with Mrs. Lewitsky and wrote a detailed note to the intern, Jeremiah, who would assume responsibility for her after me. We were never able to get her off narcotics, but we didn't really try and Dr. Cruzario never mentioned it again. As a general principle, not doing harm is a good one to remember. But it's just not that simple anymore. Harm is a multi-faceted concept and physicians regularly trade off possible harm for potential benefits in advanced medical care. The problem arises, I believe, with the *Above All* part, which oversimplifies the adage, rendering it largely useless in many real life patient situations. Mrs. Lewitsky was already an iatrogenic[vii] mess, and she was dying, alone, while we, her caretakers, had become her ersatz family, which made everything even more complicated. We don't talk much about transference and counter-transference in the ordinary doctor-patient relationship, but I suspect we should. And when a person is dying, I believed then and still believe now, she should be given the option of dying without pain. That seems the least we can do. Shouldn't the adage be *Above All, Relieve Suffering and Try Not to do Too Much Harm*?

Nowadays, pain is the fifth vital sign; we pay much more attention, though it still isn't enough. What Mrs. Lewitsky needed was palliative care, long before any such concept existed.

Two weeks later, at interns' morning report, I heard Mrs. Lewitsky had died. I had not been back to see her since I'd left her ward; I'd meant to stop in and say hello, but I never got there. She was *Do Not Resuscitate*, so no one called a code or performed CPR. She'd died alone, sometime during the night.

~

The rest of the week at Harvard Business School passed in a blur. I made no friends. I walked along the Charles each day after class, ruminating over the mess that was our health care system, running into a classmate now and again. For all my problems with cognitive dissonance, was I right in thinking that in order to solve even one problem in healthcare, we had to begin with the search for the unknown unknowns? We had to be open to the possibility that much of what we had long taken for granted wasn't just wrong; it was harmful. *Our way of thinking was harmful.* It occurred to me, in a tentative and wholly awkward way, that perhaps we needed to start changing healthcare at the end of life and work backward from there. End of life care is where most medical people have been wearing the lemon juice for too many years. We routinely make people suffer for no clear benefit except to ourselves. We don't deal with patients' fears because we harbor so much fear of our own. End of life care is filled with euphemisms and circumlocutions. In trying to treat disease and prolong life, organized medicine seems to miss the big picture. In the big picture lies the natural order of things. Our time here is limited. Nothing in medicine will ever change that.

I flew home from Cambridge and interviewed a hospital administrator. He showed me a PowerPoint presentation of his hospital's plans, based on a consultant's recent review of the marketplace. He talked about market share, competition for patients, declining revenues, payer-mixes, the importance of coding for maximum reimbursement. I'd gone directly from the theoretical to the down and dirty practical. There was not an inch of overlap, none whatsoever. How could this be? The hospital was functioning in a highly competitive environment; they were not taking the long view. They were simply a business, trying to stay afloat. He saw precisely as far as his catchment area. I felt as though I'd taken a course in macroeconomics and tried to apply the principles I'd learned to the running of a corner grocery store. One had nothing to do with the other. And yet, of course, they had everything to do with each other.

The weekend after I returned from Boston, I had twenty-four hour trauma call. One of my cases was a hip pinning in an elderly woman with advanced dementia. I walked to the waiting area to interview the patient. Her family members had gathered around the hospital bed.

I glanced through the chart then introduced myself. The patient stared straight at me, unaware, unengaged. She looked frail and tiny, but someone had carefully given her a manicure. I said hello to the family members.

One by one they introduced themselves. Mrs. J. had two daughters, a son-in-law, and a granddaughter at her bedside. I shook all their hands. I asked them questions about her medical history, about previous anesthetics, and then came to the consent form. The chart stated that Mrs. J.'s code status was *Do Not Resuscitate*.

I explained to the family that our hospital policy required us to rescind a *Do Not Resuscitate* (or *DNR* also referred to as *LET* for *Limitation of Emergency Treatment*) order for the time period that the patient is in surgery and the recovery room. I would require the signature of her power of attorney on the surgical consent form documenting this. We would reinstate the *DNR* order after the procedure was finished and Mrs. J. had returned to her room.

Mrs. J.'s daughter, Marilyn, spoke up. "I am the power of attorney, but I do not wish to change the *DNR* order. We all think it would be best for Mom if she slips away while she's under anesthesia." The family murmured their agreement, nodding.

You would not believe how many times I've had this conversation with families.

First off, this is a big area—lots of controversy and potential for change. And I get it. I wish it were that easy. I wish we had an alternative in every state to legally allow the suffering to end. But we don't. It doesn't work that way. Not yet anyway. Physician-assisted death is now legal in Washington, Oregon, Vermont, and California. Several other states have decriminalized physician-assisted suicide or have legislation under review. But this represents a very different concept from euthanasia, which is legal nowhere in the U.S. But *physician-assisted death* or *suicide* is a very different concept from *euthanasia*, which is legal nowhere. I work in Illinois—not in Switzerland, Belgium, Luxembourg, or the Netherlands. And while I stand with and applaud families for having the hard discussions and making the decisions required to be proactive with end-of-life care, the point remains that allowing a parent to "slip away" probably should not be merely an unfortunate side effect that occurs in an operating room while she's undergoing surgery for something else. Death as a *side effect* is neither a respectful treatment of a life, nor a proper use of resources. I also had to deal with my own hospital's policies.

I think this is part of the reason I suffer from cognitive dissonance. I don't know what else to call it. I empathize with these people; I have recently been in similar circumstances. We were very lucky Mom didn't have a surgical illness during the last year of her life; we did not have to make the decision quickly whether to treat or not treat. But it's not my intent to off the elderly as I go about my day job, because of insufficient discussion of what end-of-life care entails. Currently, we have no other legal mechanism in place in the hospital environment. On the other hand, people often know only what they've been told by their doctors. That is one source of my cognitive dissonance.

Patients and families do have options, though most of them do not involve institutionalized care. They don't know what they don't know. It has not been in organized medicine's best interest to tell them.

As I rolled the patient back to the operating room, I thought of a cartoon that circulated on the Internet widely a few years ago—to anesthesiologists and orthopedic surgeons alike. A cartoon orthopedic surgeon is telling an anesthesiologist that he wants to do a case. The patient is ninety-seven, in the emergency room. Healthy, he says. "There is a fracture, and I need to fix it," the cartoon orthopedic surgeon says, robotically. "Any co-morbidities?" asks the anesthesiologist, who is cute and speaks with a soft voice. "Something I have not seen before. A-sys-*tól*-e." He pronounces the word wrong. "A-sys-*tól*-e?" "Yes, a-sys-*tól*-e."

A-*SYS*-tol-e means a non-beating heart. It means the patient is dead. The surgeon wants to operate on a dead person, because the dead person has a broken bone. It's funny. Even the orthopods laugh.

# PART TWO

# Six

Dr. Robert Stein served as the Medical Examiner of Cook County from 1976 until 1993. In addition to investigating the very high profile serial killer John Wayne Gacy and the American Airlines Flight 191 crash, he gave lectures at the local Chicago area medical schools; his talks covered his specialty of forensic pathology. The two lectures he gave us, during our second year of medical school, were each about two hours in duration and were remarkable partly for the number of slide carousels that he went through during those hours and for how few people remained in the classroom at the conclusion of his talks.

~

My mother stood in the doorway to our stucco house as I exited the pink Volkswagen van that provided transportation for the Jack and Jill Nursery School in Villa Park, Illinois; it is my first clear memory of her. She asked me why I wasn't wearing a hat. Mom believed in hats. She thought cold heads resulted in head colds and nearly every ill could be prevented with a cap and muffler. She neither knew nor cared about viruses. She thought I should wear my hat even during the short walk from van to front door. I disagreed. Of course, she had been mostly deaf since shortly after birth due to the flu epidemic of 1919. But she believed she lost her hearing because of a cold breeze through an open window in the dead of winter. You don't want to argue with someone like that.

At Jack and Jill, we played musical chairs, which I loathed and which may have scarred me for life. I still worry about adequate seating. Usually some poor kid who was not paying attention got stuck without a chair. Then he stood awkwardly and felt blazingly stupid while everyone else sat comfortably and looked smug. It was a terrible game: a lesson in exclusion executed to maximize humiliation. So I drew pictures, worked with blocks, and looked forward to going home where Mom would be waiting with Oreos and milk. She always got over the hat thing.

My dad was an engineer with his own gear company; Mom stayed home with us kids. I say "us" kids, but my sisters were much older. Erica, Beth, and Bonnie were born almost exactly two years apart beginning in December 1943. More than ten years following Bonnie's birth, I arrived; they'd initially believed Mom had produced another fibroid. Later they referred to me as *the afterthought*, or sometimes as *the mistake*. Despite their ardent Catholicism, these people planned ahead. My arrival was the exception that proved the rule.

Here's what I liked from my childhood: dolls, bugs, and my sisters' math textbooks. I studied the pages of their high school geometry and algebra books as if they were illustrated bedtime stories. I couldn't understand them, but I loved the symbols, the equations, and the sharp, inky smell of the slick pages. I marveled at the smudged notations that a generation of students had illegally squiggled in the margins. I also liked piano, baseball, and the library. I suffered from severe shyness—or perhaps it wasn't shyness as much as *otherness*, a sense of being apart—so solitary pursuits suited me perfectly. As a result, I read a wide variety of non-juvenile and surprisingly helpful self-help material. For example, I was deathly afraid of the dentist. I speculated that if I didn't smile, my parents would forget I had teeth. This actually worked. I managed to go years without a dental check-up, pulling out my own teeth as necessary. Fortunately, I never had a cavity.

After three daughters, my parents admitted they wanted a boy. Once they'd had me—a non-boy—they kept talking about it. My mother often said out loud: "Gosh darn it, I wanted a red-headed boy just like my brother Johnny!" They couldn't let it go. So they tried to make me look like a boy. I'm sure this was unconscious on their parts, but it confused me nonetheless. I felt strangely neutered and self-conscious. In grade school, I had straight white hair cut short by an unsmiling German lady with rice pudding arms who worked at a salon near our house. She terrified me with her guttural accent and glinting scissors. Dad abetted this situation by explaining all about Nazi Germany, torture, and the concentration camps. He went on about the Holocaust and Nuremburg Trials, the Berlin Wall, East and West Germany, the Stasi secret police, and I got the point. I knew—with the grave certainty that exemplified my childhood—this transplanted woman would cut off my ear if I didn't sit perfectly still. Each time, in the car going to the beauty salon, I begged my mother to please make the German lady leave the bangs a little bit longer. I hated it when strangers—at Baskin-Robbins or the post office—called me "son"; I wanted to cry. Once I stuffed my shirt with Kleenex but my sister Bonnie laughed and told her friends.

We lived in an excellent neighborhood, filled with big families, lots of kids my age, and old people. I missed having grandparents so I frequently visited the neighbors'. I liked that they stayed home in the afternoons when I came to call. I felt comfortable with old people; I enjoyed sitting with them, playing card games, swapping stories. Two doors away the Feulners had a grandmother who was stout like pictures of the sepia-colored ancestors hanging on our living room walls. But she smiled and gave out cookies. I figured the women in the pictures probably did that too, just assumed harsh poses for the portraits. If I ever had my portrait taken, I planned to look quite severe. And down the block on the other side was a great-grandmother who was the oldest person alive. She didn't see well, so I read to her sometimes. I remember when she turned one hundred—her family put up a large sign in their front yard. When her cat had kittens, her daughter let me visit every day. I loved the kittens—my family considered themselves dog people—but I preferred talking to the delicate and shrunken woman who had the amazing freedom to say out loud what the rest of us were thinking. It seemed to me that speech wasn't really free; it came with a terrible price—like dependence and canes and sometimes smelling bad. I thought older people should get more perks, should demand more respect for their wisdom, more deference for their hard-earned paradigm shift. You shouldn't have to go through eighty or eighty-five years before you had a screened-in porch from which to view the yard and flowers, to keep the bugs out and the cats in while enjoying a good sit. You shouldn't have to wait until everyone had stopped listening before you got to say what was really on your mind.

When I was a first-grader, Mom took classes in lip-reading. Each night we watched Walter Cronkite deliver the evening news with the sound off. She had, as she called them, "one good ear and one bad ear". The bad ear was completely deaf. The good ear tended to go bad in the winter. Though she lost her hearing at age two, it was many years before anyone figured it out. Without basic medical care and visual or auditory screening, she had been placed in the back of the classroom along with the other "imbeciles". She was told she was stupid and she believed it. Mom dropped out of school in eighth grade. During the Depression, her family needed whatever money she could contribute. She babysat for local children and worked on farms during the summer months. My grandfather—whose family had disowned him when he married my grandmother—had died during the flu epidemic that took Mom's hearing in 1919, leaving grandma Nellie alone with five kids, ages fourteen to two. She cleaned houses to make ends meet, as it were. After Nellie's father passed in 1920, food grew scarce and they often survived on potatoes. Mom's sister Fern contracted rheumatic fever. Nellie herself became ill. At one particularly low point, the State of Illinois took Fern and Johnny away from Nellie, placing them in an orphanage for a time. Mom, as the youngest, was allowed to stay with her mother. Her sister Martha and brother James were just old enough to fend for themselves. Martha and Johnny both contracted TB; only Martha survived. Johnny died when Mom was nineteen.

So I didn't argue with the lip-reading lessons. I rarely argued with her at all. In general I got along really well with my mother except that she wanted me to be an extrovert, which I wasn't. That problem caused the most conflict between us. She wanted me to socialize in a way that was as inconceivable to me at age six or twelve as it is to me today. My mother thought that by signing me up for every lesson available to a child in Elmhurst, I could overcome my shyness and introversion. As a result, I took horseback riding, printmaking, tennis, golf, piano, racquetball, photography lessons; you name it and I took a lesson in it. None of the lessons changed my personality, however. As a child, I was much as I am now. Smaller, perhaps, and willing to eat fewer vegetables. I was born quiet with a tendency to stay off to the side, pay attention, and learn. Just like my mom. And after observing my sisters' adolescences, I saw the value in flying under the radar; I made it a habit that served me well.

~

Dr. Stein was not a particularly eloquent speaker. I recall his voice as raspy, his manner as gruff. The power of his delivery lay not in the words he chose to describe his work; rather, the power lay in the images depicted by the slides that were projected onto the screen in the front of our very ordinary classroom. He explained how he gathered clues from the circumstances and the wounds to determine the cause and the time of death—it all seemed relatively straightforward, if you had the stomach for it. But these weren't the types of deaths I'd ever heard about it before, and certainly never since. These weren't the kinds of deaths you see on *Law and Order*, even the *Special Victims Unit*. These were homicides of such atrocity, such depravity, that I could never speak of them again. And there were dozens. He cleared the room with his stories and pictures of death. There were only a handful of us remaining after four hours with Dr. Stein. It didn't occur to me to wonder—at the time—why

I stayed and listened and watched while Dr. Stein gave us his lectures on forensic pathology. I am not a fan of horror. I do not go to scary movies; I do not read frightening books.

~

Being the youngest by a decade gave me an interesting perspective. My parents and sisters constituted a family of their own; I watched them interact with a curious detachment. I studied the dynamics created by my father's ambition and hard work, his overriding sense of obligation, his occasional fits of rage, and the brilliant dispassion he could bring to difficult topics. My mother worshipped him; he was her lost father, her lost brother, her partner, and her lover. He valued her tough common sense, her intelligence, and her convert's zealous faith. He relied heavily on her unwavering support; only she could point out his mistakes and get away with it. He was, by far, the more emotional of the two. They worked in synchrony together, understanding perfectly each other's strengths and limitations. And when they fought, they argued over some edict of my father's; his autocratic manner sat poorly with my rational, democratic mom. I have many memories of her holding up a fist behind his back.

My parents believed they were incredibly lucky, and knew that luck often depended on the kindness of others. They gave charitably of their time as well as their money. Mom hired women who lived in the worst of Chicago's housing projects. She helped them in a variety of ways—money, clothing, food. Then she made my father drive them home when they left our house after dark, even in the late sixties during the Democratic National Convention. I remember the fear on his face to this day. She hired the handicapped: our housepainter had five fingers total—on both hands. One cleaning lady was a paranoid schizophrenic who plainly terrified Dad. Mom worked with psych patients, and when I was a young teen, she took me with her: we played golf with the inpatients at the Hines VA Hospital on the three-hole course. She delivered Meals-on-Wheels for decades. And at many times during my childhood and adolescence we had someone living in our basement—some guy who was temporarily out of work or needed a helping hand for a few months to get through a rough spot. Dad would periodically show up with a car he'd bought from someone who needed to sell something. Men would appear to do work on our house or our yard—men who were down on their luck. Then they would disappear. And reappear for Thanksgiving dinner.

I don't know where my interest in medicine came from; my parents never encouraged me in any particular direction. Dad tended to avoid visiting sick friends until the stink of infirmity had left them. Once when I was twelve years old, he took me along to see his friend Sam in the hospital. Sam had been an original investor in the gear company and he'd suffered a heart attack. A surprising number of Dad's friends—men from his Pot Luck Group, neighbors, as well as acquaintances from the gear business—had died suddenly from heart disease. I remember Sam's face, normally tanned from exhaustive golf, looking pale against the hospital bed. An oxygen cannula hooked around both ears and across his face like a plastic moustache. Dad pressed a kiss to Sam's forehead, then sat beside his bed. I sat behind him on the radiator cover.

"I need to tell you a story," Sam said. His voice seemed clear and strong. I felt relieved. I didn't want him to be sick. He had a son my age.

"Anything," Dad replied.

"I guess my heart stopped a few times."

Dad nodded.

"I want you to remember what I'm going to tell you. I'm afraid I'll forget. I don't want to forget this."

He wiped carefully at the corners of his mouth with a Kleenex.

"I could see them working on me. Could hear them. It's like I was above them, floating, in a corner of the room. And I watched, but I kept drifting away. I saw a bright light, and I moved toward it through a dark tunnel, but then I was watching again. They were pushing on my chest."

Dad turned and met my eyes, to make certain I was paying attention. I shook my head slightly to indicate my amazement.

"I won't forget," Dad said. Then he asked, "Was there pain?"

Sam shook his head, and closed his eyes.

"I won't forget," Dad repeated. And neither did I. These were the early days of CPR.

~

I think it was near the end of the two lectures, after four hours of Dr. Stein's horror show, that he uttered the words that stayed with me forever. All those slides, the many carousels, the endless supply of images, had all come out of the Cook County Medical Examiner's office in the prior *six months*. It seemed as though it could have been a lifetime of misery, a career's worth of atrocity. But all those events had occurred in just the previous half year.

I realized then the enormity of what I didn't know. Usually when I had similar thoughts, they felt humbling and vaguely educational. *Margaret, see how much you have to learn.* But isn't that good? As though more knowledge will make me better, richer somehow, and more well rounded. After those lectures I knew, in my heart, that I didn't know and *could not imagine* what I didn't know. I was not better for it. I might have felt safer. But I was not, in fact, safer.

~

"Margaret," my mother called to me from the kitchen one evening. We lived in a well-maintained two-story stucco home on the edge of Elmhurst College. We had a smallish garden that steadfastly refused to grow anything besides spindly pink roses. I had planted assorted vegetables throughout my childhood and adolescence. They all proved inedible. I think we had bad soil. "Where are you going this evening?"

At seventeen, I had several diverse groups of friends, a few of which liked to party. I often bought beer from two brothers who owned a liquor store on a corner about six blocks from my house and who didn't card. The older brother, Doug, had a wife and a baby and didn't flirt as much as his younger sibling. Jeremy was the cute one. I made certain I wore tight jeans, a t-shirt, no bra, and smiled a lot. I looked about fourteen. Never once did I have to show my fake ID. The guys in our group supplied the weed. I never asked where they got it. Every weekend we smoked and drank. It was the seventies.

"Mom," I said, "I'm going to drink alcohol and smoke marijuana tonight."

"Oh you are not. What are really going to do?"

"I just told you. I'm going to Dolly's house and we're all getting *smashed* and watching *Monty Python*."

"Oh, you. Be home by midnight. You know I don't sleep until I hear you come in."

So I partied, and my mom pretended she didn't know. Maybe she didn't. I maintained straight A's; that was the important thing. I think my parents were worn out. They were in their mid-fifties by the time I started high school and, having grown up during the Depression, they'd suffered through every hardship already. My dad raised plenty of hell in his time; nothing I could ever do would surprise him. And they were sick and tired of parenting. They thought of me as being utterly responsible, so they just figured I was smart enough not to screw it up. They counted on it. What surprised the hell out of me was that they were right.

Sometime in high school, I decided to become a doctor—quite possibly a psychiatrist. I thought every family should have one so I nominated myself. I'd read that medicine was a recession-proof industry. And I might get to save lives, or something of that nature, which seemed like a good idea at the time. My parents supported this decision, insofar as they understood it. My dad didn't exactly approve of medicine as a career choice; unless you manufactured a product, in his view, you weren't contributing to society. With that encouragement I left nothing to chance and interviewed—at seventeen—for med school. I'd found an accelerated program. My mother had begun attending Mass daily, praying fervently for my acceptance.

After a few generalities, the surgeon who conducted the interview asked, "Why should we spend all this time and money educating you when you'll probably just quit and have babies?"

As a teenager, babies were nowhere on my agenda, but I'd heard I might be asked the question. I had embraced feminism in fifth grade. During the seventies, when some of us still hoped for the ratification of the Equal Rights Amendment, men asked questions like this. (Now, well so much has changed, hasn't it?) After a moment, I said to the surgeon, "I don't see why I can't practice medicine and have a family too." I don't know what answer he expected, but that one proved sufficient. They let me in. I figured that whatever I was getting into, I'd somehow make it work. My mother had told me that I could be whatever I wanted to be. While I suspected that wasn't entirely true—I thought it would be cool to be a flight surgeon or a jet pilot but they weren't hiring women—it seemed true enough.

The questions I considered during the nine months at Harvard Business School were neither new nor original. But their context had simultaneously grown in scope and narrowed in focus. They were, essentially, the questions of my youth and young adulthood; in my family, we discussed these issues over breakfast, over popcorn snacks in the afternoon, and over leisurely dinners. It was only after many years and after both Mom and Dad had passed that I recognized the significance of the questions and those early conversations. Until I left home,

I thought the conversations of our household—about personal responsibility, about preparation for old age and dying—were routine. I learned, over the span of my career, that they were anything but common and the principles evoked were incendiary to some, painful to others. Though my parents disparaged, if they even entertained, the concept of exceptionalism, especially *American exceptionalism*, they were exceptional *in this way*. My father spoke often, even *ad nauseam*, of his eventual death. We made fun of him for it. We hung dishrags over his portrait in the living room, goading him. We rolled our eyes as he brought up yet another discussion of advance directives, before advance directives had a name. Of course we didn't want to hear about his death planning; we were his kids. But slowly, eventually, we came to understand. The idea of planning for the inevitable is not that you can control what ultimately happens to you, but that the more preparation you have, the fewer surprises will await you and your loved ones. Why did he believe that? I don't know. He was smarter than me. He knew that life deals whatever blows it will; nothing will change that simple fact. Preparation allows us to handle adversity with added dexterity.

~

Dr. Stein's lectures were my first experience with learning about the unknown unknowns. The horrors that were part of his everyday life were completely foreign to me. And they would be foreign to almost everyone I know. They fall outside the realm of what seems reasonable and right.

There was no planning for the victims in the slides Stein showed us, in the stories he told. They died sudden and violent deaths. For those tragic people, preparation was a luxury denied.

# Seven

Imagine you are a medical doctor; it is a very odd thing to be. People—usually strangers—take off their clothes for you, let you touch their skin and see them naked. You examine their orifices, listen to their bodily functions, then fill them with potentially toxic chemicals. They tell you their secrets when you've only just met. You do not reciprocate.

It takes chutzpah to be a doctor. It requires something like courage or astonishing insensitivity to invade privacy to the extent that you do, to invade the boundaries of normal interpersonal relationships. It takes a strong stomach, a poker face, and an ability to think on your feet. A sense of humor helps enormously because people can be very odd.

Patients may hate you while holding you in the highest esteem. They hate the intimacy of your relationship with them; they hate the power they must give up to you and your ability to make mistakes at their expense. They hate that you charge them for services that hold no guarantees and that may actually cause them harm. You cannot blame them for that. Conversely, they may think you are terrific when you are not, in fact, terrific in the least. They do not have to know you or your skills in order to think these things.

Medical school makes you tough and residency makes you tougher. So tough, in fact, that your own friends and family cannot stand you sometimes. When did that happen? How tough you get—or how jaded or how 'anesthetized' to your work—is not determined by a single event, or patient, or book, or any given teacher. It's determined by all of those and more. It's determined by who you are when you start and the role models you meet, whether you're looking for them or not. It's easy, in fact, to get too tough: imagine real life in a pot, simmered hours too long, until its essence is thick, juices evaporated, just tough meat remaining. Take out the joy, the insulation of social conventions, leave the chronicity of sickness and death, add stress, plus a healthy dose of fear. Then call it a career.

When you get an MD, you receive some amazing privileges. But there are no guarantees of either empathy or compassion. You can be kind or a jerk or both, sometimes within a single hour of a single day. Because it is a strange thing that you do—few other professions compare. Unfortunately, when you do it over the course of years, you forget how strange it is. *You forget how privileged you are.* You lose your perspective. Many practitioners never get it back. Most never get it back.

Medical students decide on a specialty during their third and fourth years of medical school. I wanted to love psychiatry, but didn't. The psychiatrists I met seemed disconnected, unhappy, or flamboyantly odd. I also realized I suffered from severe motion sickness, which meant certain specialties were out of the question. Anything involving a moving screen or a microscope made me nauseous—so pathology, ophthalmology, and radiology were disqualified. I spent a day with a pediatrician in the suburbs and nearly dropped dead from boredom. I considered internal medicine and, one-by-one, all of the subspecialties but none of the organ systems caught my interest. I felt lost and tried to determine which group of doctors seemed normal, or most like me. Was I normal?

I knew of one here, one there. Not so many, really. No obvious clusters. So many people seemed kinda sorta unhappy. Did I want to be a doctor?

There was also the matter of getting unexpectedly pregnant at the age of twenty-four during my last year of medical school. I had six months to choose a specialty in which I could manage motherhood as well.

Then during my obstetrical rotation, a third year anesthesia resident named Ron Meyer went out of his way to teach me about anesthesiology, about labor and delivery, about the equipment. He was serious, likable, meticulous, and he loved what he did. He actively recruited me into the specialty. *We relieve pain and people hardly ever die in anesthesia*, he said. *And new safety devices are constantly being developed, so even fewer will die in the future. It's a great specialty.* I liked this idea of nobody dying. *You'd be good at this*, he said. Nobody had said that before. They proved to be powerful words. And most of the anesthesiologists I met seemed very calm: compared to internists and pediatricians they had a sense of humor, and compared to surgeons they seemed humble humanitarians. I liked the OR vibe. As a group, anesthesiologists were nerdy but companionable. Like me. They had perspective and a reasonable view of the human condition. I could make it work with motherhood, I hoped. So I signed up.

My dad was disappointed when I told him I had decided to go into anesthesiology. I think it was the word—anesthesiologist—with its odd combination of syllables and consonants. He said it made him lisp. The operating room was a world he could not—or would not—fathom. But I also think he had an old-fashioned idea of what doctors should be, drawn from Norman Rockwell paintings and *Marcus Welby* shows. He thought of doctors as kindly souls with starched gray coats who made house calls and had babies named after them. That had been my idea too—I'd grown up with a crush on Chad Everett from *Medical Center*—but medicine was highly sub-specialized by the time I arrived. Dad could not fit that image together with me working in an operating room.

When I told my mother of my chosen field, she said, "Oh, honey, I don't think that's such a good idea. Won't you be on your feet a lot?" I laughed at the time, but she was right as usual.

~

Eighteen months later I was a brand new anesthesia resident carrying the cardiac arrest pager for the first time. I clipped the pager to my waist, where it pulled at the drawstring of my scrub pants like a live grenade. When it started to chirp, just moments

71

after it was passed to me at our local VA hospital, I heard a simultaneous overhead page to a *code blue* on the fifth floor. I ran up three flights of stairs, down a long hall, and arrived in single room—heart pounding and out of breath. As the anesthesia resident on call, it was my responsibility to put breathing tubes into the windpipes of the nearly departed, a process referred to as intubation, an essential skill of anesthesiologists everywhere. I stood at the head of the bed and remembered that very morning when a venerable professor had said to me, "You can't intubate the broad side of a barn!" He'd observed me under the best of all possible circumstances, in an operating room, with a completely anesthetized, fully paralyzed patient without teeth to obstruct my vision. He was correct. I had no skills. Now everyone at this poor patient's cardiac arrest would learn the truth.

~

Every day for forty-five years, my father timed his four and a half mile drive to and from work. He tried every route, every conceivable combination of streets, and kept track of how long each trip took. He knew the duration of every green/yellow/red light because he kept track. He knew how many cars could make a left hand turn onto northbound Route 83 from eastbound North Avenue; he calculated the average length of each car and average distance between the cars. The radio, he said, distracted him from problem solving. He hated to drive and he hated waiting. Timing different routes satisfied the mathematician in him and made the time pass.

Dad was born in Paris, Texas, but grew up in Chicago. His mother, Clara, came from Burlington, Wisconsin where her family had settled in the mid-eighteen hundreds. Clara married Platte Overton—eleven years her junior—when she was in her late thirties; he was the eldest son in a family of twelve and a heating and air-conditioning engineer who wrote a textbook on forced air heating in 1934. Platte had a wandering eye. My grandparents officially split up when Dad was a young teen, but Platte had been no more than an intermittent presence. Dad saw his father once in my lifetime—I believe they went thirty-eight years between visits—and I never met my grandfather. Platte remarried, moved to California, and forgot about his first family. My grandfather's very existence was something we didn't discuss; he had abandoned Dad as well as his brother, Platte Jr., who was mentally handicapped. I don't think I even knew I had a living grandfather until I was twelve. I also didn't know that I had an aunt—my father had a full sister—who came along before Clara and Platte had married. Born in 1914, Aunt Betty was sent away to Seattle to be raised by a childless couple. Dad and Betty finally met when they were both in their sixties; together they concluded that she'd had the better childhood. My dad was able to get to know Betty and her family before she died of renal failure a few years later.

~

The veteran lying before me did not look well. Two weeks into anesthesia residency and even I could see it. Which made perfect sense, seeing as how technically he was dead. But a code had been called because he had been found without a pulse, not breathing, and he did not have a *Do Not Resuscitate* order. Completely emaciated, probably from cancer, he couldn't have weighed more than eighty pounds. A male medical student performed CPR and since the patient had a feeding tube, which no one had bothered to discontinue, every time the student pushed down on the chest a fresh wave of Vanilla Ensure gurgled backwards through the patient's nose. Every other compression or so, the dull crack of another rib cut through the sounds of the ECG machine which registered artifact in sporadic beeps and hisses.

~

My grandma Clara had two spinster sisters—Kate and Nora Wagner—who lived in Burlington, Wisconsin in the family home until the early seventies, when I was a young teen. Kate and Nora—ancient and good-natured—lived for gossip and my father's visits. On Sunday afternoons, we would sit in the white wicker rocking chairs in the sunny end of the old dining room with its pressed tin ceiling and glass cabinets and I would study a math textbook, then carefully go exploring. I particularly loved the kitchen with its cracked linoleum, ancient sink, and nineteen-twenties stove. Off the porch was a large stone where, in the days before cars, you stood to climb onto your horse or into your buggy.

Across the alley lay the Burlington police station, and on the opposite side of the house where there was once a vineyard, a gas station had been built. My great-grandfather had owned the local hardware store, and a long dead great-uncle and his sons had started a foundry behind the old house; they manufactured bullrings and calf-weaners. I always imagined calf-weaners were somehow attached to the cow, like cruel and radical nipple piercing. It wasn't until my dad was gone and my mom came to stay with me that she explained: a calf-weaner is a metal or plastic device affixed to a calf's lip or nose that prevents it from sucking, in order to wean a calf from its mother's teat. Wagner bullrings and calf-weaners are still made, though the company was sold long ago. My great-uncle Charles Wagner patented the self-piercing bullring on December 19th, 1916 that is still in production. I feel curiously proud of this fact.

~

For my part in the code blue, I held a mask over the patient's face. This was no simple task what with the Ensure and all, and periodically I tried to get his jaw open in order to insert the laryngoscope and intubate his trachea. But the jaw was clenched tight. Having been told that very morning that I couldn't intubate

74

a barn, I assumed my inability to open the fellow's mouth arose from my own incompetence and even if I had been able to get into his mouth, I wouldn't have been able to see anything but Ensure. I decided to try to nasally intubate. I stuffed a smallish tube through the left nare and shoved blindly, thinking, what the hell, maybe I'll get lucky and this thing will slip miraculously into the windpipe. But that didn't work. I didn't feel well. The smell of Ensure was making me gag. This poor man was barely more than a carcass, a skeleton. Perhaps irrationally, I felt as though it was all my fault that we couldn't revive him. And yet, realistically, I was too inexperienced to think realistically.

~

Each week, weather permitting, we took Kate and Nora to the cemetery to visit the family's graves. I liked studying the headstones and wondering what might have caused the people, particularly the infants, to die. I liked the cemetery in general—it sat on a hill on the outskirts of town and afforded a pleasant view. It seemed a good spot to spend an afternoon and, possibly, eternity. I thought to myself: *this is what old people do. They visit graves. They grow facial hair and drink Riesling. They read books from the library. Not bad.* My dad told me that Nora had dated Babe Ruth—she'd been a looker in her day. Later I was disappointed to learn that Babe wasn't all that particular.

Dad credited the Boy Scouts for saving him from a life of "debauchery" and turning him into a responsible and moral person. A Catholic priest led the troop and served as his role model. Dad attended Chicago's Crane High School. From there he was accepted into a work/study program at Armor Institute with his best friend, Warren Hutchins. They had competed for the same scholarship, but ultimately the program decided to award two, one to each of them. Dad and Hutch worked together for five decades. Armor later became Illinois Institute of Technology, and they worked at the Illinois Gear Company for a number of years. They learned all about the manufacturing and sales of precision gears, which were used in locomotive engines, army tanks, and so on.

~

One of the senior residents arrived at the code. A tall slender woman with dark brown hair, Anna had been my supervisor for one month during internship. She taught me everything I knew about ordering out for pizza on call nights. She taught me nothing else.

~

George Sullivan fixed up my parents on a blind date in the summer of *1938*. They ate dinner at the Edgewater Beach Hotel in Chicago, a famous and posh and pink north side landmark that was demolished in 1967. The hotel was known for the stars it attracted and the bands it hosted, like Tommy Dorsey and Glenn Miller. A friend of mine heard Frank Sinatra sing there once—he casually performed for the crowd while sipping a drink at the bar. Frank wasn't that type of guy ordinarily, but The Edgewater was that kind of place. It was love at first sight for Lydia and Carl. They married in 1941.

Dad took a job at Brad Foote Gear after Illinois Gear fired him. There, he negotiated with union representatives on behalf of the management. Those were turbulent times in labor relations and he carried a gun for a while. He left Brad Foote to start his own gear manufacturing company (with Hutch and six other investors) in Chicago's western suburbs in 1955. It seemed risky. He had a wife, three kids, a mother, and a handicapped brother to support. But he recognized opportunity. He knew he had to take a risk to get ahead. And he understood the benefit of having been fired *once*. "Make your failures count, Margaret." He told me it had prompted soul-searching and created a learning experience that persistent success could never duplicate.

~

"How long has he been down?" Anna asked the junior resident running the code.

"At least 20 minutes," he answered. "That's when he was found."

"Can't get a tube in him?" she asked me.

"No," I said. "Can't get his mouth open."

She stepped up to the side of the bed, picked up the patient's arm, tried to bend it at the elbow. When it didn't bend, she dropped it back onto the bed.

~

Dad had an obsessive interest in end-of-life planning. He did everything he could, from a legal standpoint, to organize. He had a living will and a healthcare power of attorney long before anyone else I'd known or heard about. He thought it all through. Dad liked to discuss other topics—like golf, politics, history, and religion—but he rarely let an opportunity pass where he failed to mention something related to death, possibly his own or perhaps the recent deaths of people he knew. He taught me to read the obituaries from a very young age. He utilized every family gathering as an opportunity to discuss some aspect of his ultimate demise: his will, estate planning, trust, educational generation-skipping trust, power of attorney, advance directives, and other similar topics. He believed in planning even for things you can't really plan for, because he saw the value in thinking through a variety of possible, even improbable, scenarios. It seemed more than a little morbid. But he possessed great mental agility that allowed him to imagine not just one or two sides to any given issue, but multiple sides. And that ability never rendered him indecisive. He sent us photocopies of handwritten letters that began "Dear E/B/B/M," updating us on changes or corrections to the needlessly complex documents undergoing constant revision by an attorney even older than he. These letters predated the forms for advance directives that you can download off the Internet today. They predated the Internet. He left nothing to chance. He kept his family close because he knew we'd be the ones to take care of him in the end. He didn't want to be institutionalized. He wanted to die at home. He wanted to be with family and in control. He had a fear of hospitals and of nursing homes which was, in retrospect, healthy. He knew that you reap what you sow.

One day he sent us a convoluted rationale that explained why he should only fly first class. He was in his seventies. He presented his calculations, figuring in how much money would go to charity and estate taxes, concluding that it would cost each one of us an additional $1.35 for every trip he took in first class as opposed to coach. He'd already told me—on multiple occasions—never to trust an accountant, so I didn't believe him for a moment. He could crunch numbers to make anything seem either completely reasonable or utterly ludicrous. Guys like that usually work for the Government Accounting Office.

~

"Let's call this code," Anna said, looking at her watch. "It's 3:30. Stop chest compressions, turn off the EKG. Stop the IV's." She stepped back from the bed, hands on hips, and shook her head. "This patient is dead. And he has been dead at least 6 hours. You can't open the mouth because rigor mortis has set in." She paused, searched our faces, then said, "Didn't anyone notice that this man is room temperature?"

# Eight

Scientists at the Mayo Clinic have genetically engineered mice to age five times more quickly than normal. These special mice lack a protein that the investigators have labeled *BubR1*. Consequently, the mice develop cataracts, hunched spines, and produce high levels of a tumor-suppressing molecule called *p16Ink4a*, known as "p16" for short. This molecule in and of itself accelerates cellular senescence in more normal lab mice.

~

I had two job offers when I finished anesthesia residency. The one I didn't take was in a Chicago department run by an Iranian guy who'd had a facelift and wore a toupee. He called me Dolores and offered the job to my breasts; the four of us declined the position. It wasn't that the other job offered more money, I told my parents, even though that had something to do with it. No, I told them. I chose to work at this large suburban trauma center not far from their house based on the quality of the candy sold in the gift shop. Since they shared my sweet tooth, they understood. Every occasion in my family prompted a trip to the Fannie Mae store in Elmhurst. Birthdays, Easter, Mother's Day, Fourth of July, even Groundhog Day provided my parents with a reason to shop for sweets. When Bea was born during my last year of medical school, Dad brought a five-pound box of Pixies to the maternity ward. When Ruthann came along during third year of residency, I received two pounds of Frango Mints. So it seemed natural that I chose the job with the best candy selection. *They stocked Bun candy bars!* Not only did I have a reliable source of Buns, Caramel Creams, Twizzlers, and bite-size Reese's Peanut Butter Cups, but my parents lived nearby. They could help me with childcare when necessary, which they did frequently, generously and without complaint. My family had no idea what I did for a living, but they were proud of me in the abstract. And they adored their grandchildren.

As the only physician in the family, I became the go-to person for all medical matters. We have been, for most of our lives, a remarkably healthy bunch. I have studied my ancestry on both sides and people have lived into the nineties for generations. Personally, I don't want to live into my nineties. Between my mom and my grandmother, I'm pretty sure I'll have dementia. It's the curse of good genes. I'll have my dad's bad joints and my mother's bad brain. What to do? I could take my therapist's cue and buy a gun. Only based on my experiences at the hospital, seeing the patients I've seen, I'd probably just blow off an ear or shoot myself in the foot. Anyway, my parents loved to ask my advice for problems large and small, but they rarely followed it.

A typical case of the stomach flu went like this: Carl would call and say, "Your mother has the runs. What should we do?"

"Tell her to have only clear liquids today. Chicken broth, tea, Jell-O."

"What kind of Jell-O?" he would ask, as if it mattered.

"Whatever kind of Jell-O she likes."

Then he would interrupt and talk to my mother. "What kind of Jell-O do you like, honey? Maybe I'd better look to see what we have. Your mother says we have cherry."

"Dad..."

"I see some cherry here in the cabinet. There's strawberry too. Which one is better, do you think?"

"Dad! It doesn't matter. The point is to give her some hydration, as long as she isn't vomiting. Whatever type of Jell-O you've got is fine. And no food until the diarrhea starts to slow down."

"Oh. Okay, thanks."

"Then tomorrow, if it's better, you can start her on the BRAT diet," I would say. "That's an acronym for bananas, rice, applesauce and toast. Are you writing this down? Basically, keep it bland until she's having formed stools. Any fever?"

"No, I don't think so." He covered the mouthpiece and yelled at Mom to inquire about her fever. "No, no fever."

We typically had the same conversation two or three times a year, as if it had never occurred before. And each time it came as a surprise to my parents that cottage cheese, fresh fruit, ice cream, and a nice Michigan Riesling were not the cure that they'd hoped for their bowel problems.

Often they would call with questions about friends' medical conditions and prognoses, or tell horror stories about medical care gotten "elsewhere". I would listen attentively, make suggestions, even offer to help them get in touch with a physician. Each time they asked for advice for themselves, they would seem to listen, say "Oh, *real*-ly," with apparent appreciation, then basically ignore everything I'd said. Sometimes Dad would call and ask my then-husband for his advice, which I found particularly annoying until I realized that he ignored that too. These phone calls were so frequent that I came to regard them as routine, insignificant, and rather tiresome. That is, until the day the call came that caught me off guard. That was the one that actually mattered.

~

Cellular senescence means that cells stop dividing; they get *old*. Senescent cells actually accumulate in human beings as well as in genetically engineered mice.[ix] Imagine the implications. Someday there might be drugs to slow the damage wrought by certain types of painful arthritis.

~

The phone rang on a day when I was at home, resting, after trauma call. It was a particularly warm afternoon in late January 1997.

My parents had recently returned from a trip to Kenya and

Tanzania where they'd been on a photo safari. Dad showed me a picture Mom had taken of him with a Masai warrior who stood a full foot taller. He said they'd talked about women, about their wives in particular. The warrior had four. My dad said he could barely handle my mother.

"Is this Doctor Overton?" a voice asked.

My parents seemed older but not old at seventy-nine. Mom walked every day and did yoga. Dad still worked, swam a mile four days a week, golfed poorly and often. But since their return from Africa, he hadn't been feeling well. So he'd gone to Rochester for the three-day executive physical. He'd done this in the past, and loved telling a story about having trouble with an ankle a couple years earlier. He'd flown up to Minnesota, checked in to the World Famous Mayo Clinic, and undergone the usual battery of rigorous tests. The Mayo doctors told him to take two ibuprofen and put his foot up. He thought that was hilarious. Such prestige, such wealth of knowledge, and they recommended *Motrin*.

"Yes. I'm Margaret Overton."

"My name is Alan Adams. I was asked to see your dad because of a spot on his lung that showed up on an X-ray. We've done a CT scan of his chest, and it doesn't look like there's any evidence of spread, but I believe he should be operated on, to have this removed. It is likely to be malignant."

"He never smoked," I said. I felt dumb. My first thought was that my dad couldn't have lung cancer. Other people smoked, but not him. He took care of himself. I'd forgotten that it's all a crapshoot. People just get what they get.

"That's what he said. This is probably an adenocarcinoma. We were discussing where your father should have this done, and we would be happy to do his surgery here, but he wanted to discuss it with you first."

"Okay. Thanks. Can you put my dad on?"

Dad's voice returned to the line. "Yeah," he said briskly, "do you want to think it over and call me back?"

It wasn't necessary. One of our closest friends was an excellent thoracic surgeon. "Come home, we'll take care of it here, Dad. Dave can do the surgery. It will be much easier on Mom if you're close by. Easier for all of us."

"That's what I was thinking too. But I wondered, is this difficult surgery? I mean, should I have another opinion, look around for the most experienced surgeon?"

"Dave is very competent; the group does a lot of thoracic surgery. You'll be in good hands," I said. "This should be pretty straightforward."

"Right. Talk to you later." I heard the click at the other end, then silence.

I looked down at the phone in my hand. *Straightforward*, I'd told him. My dad had lung cancer and I casually told him it should be straightforward. Nice work, Margaret.

~

Dr. Jan van Deursen is a Mayo scientist in the field of aging, and one of the authors of a paper that was published in 2011 titled "Clearance of p16Ink4a-positive senescent cells delays ageing-associated disorders," which appeared in the journal *Nature*. He and his group of researchers designed an animal model—the BubR1 deficient mouse—from which he could easily clear senescent cells to see what happened. And what happened was this: after injecting his mice with a particular chemical known as AP20187, his aging mice didn't get cataracts, or muscle wasting, or lose subcutaneous fat. His mice didn't get wrinkles. His treated progeroid[x] mice ("progeroid" refers to premature aging) didn't need Botox or joint replacements.

~

I sat on the edge of a chaise lounge and gazed out at my back yard, at the zip line that my dog loved, at the swing set the kids had outgrown. And I wondered: when exactly did my parents morph from solid and sturdy to not-quite-frail, but vulnerable? On one hand, they were always a little older. They were over forty when they had me. On the other hand, they were active, constantly traveling or playing golf; they were not sedentary people. When I was thirty, we took a trip together to Brazil. They left me in Sao Paulo; I went home and they took a boat up the Amazon River. This adventurous pair took trips all the time: pilgrimages, safaris—they saw the *Passion Play* in Oberammergau, they travelled to Lourdes and Medjugorje. Dad still worked full-time.

So even though they grew older before my eyes, I didn't really see it; they didn't act old. The aging process seemed slow, imperceptible even, except—now that I thought about it—I guess Dad's handwriting had started to look a bit craggy. I remembered another day I noticed he'd missed a spot shaving, then a week later he missed the same spot. What was that about? My mother never aged at all except that she inexplicably took to wearing jeans and plaid flannel shirts every day after a lifetime of following fashion. Gradually Dad seemed more consistently irascible, but hadn't he always sort of been that way? Perhaps aging slowly peeled back a lid, which allowed his ornery but true self to escape from the dampening effect of social pressures. Occasionally he did goofy things but they typically involved driving. He'd always been a terrible driver so it wasn't unusual for him to tear through a construction site or rip the drainpipe off the side of the house with his bumper. He treated his car more as a tractor than a luxury vehicle.

And then one day—maybe it was that day, sitting there on that stupid lounge chair on which one could neither properly sit nor lounge, talking to a surgeon at the Mayo Clinic—it hit me that this road was *one way*. They were further along than I realized, and they weren't coming back from this aging thing. I depended on them for so much—I called my mom before I called anyone. I didn't fully appreciate her until the day I gave birth to Bea and then I realized she knew everything. Dad and I had a tug-of-war over her after that, which he won, naturally. And as for him, I could always count on my father for an objective assessment of a difficult problem. He might be temperamental or ornery or occasionally explosive, but I knew I could depend on him to do the right thing. My parents were smart and loving and had my best interests at heart. They helped with my kids whenever I asked. They would come home from Florida if I needed them. They didn't make me crazy. They were good to me. I saw that gradually, over time, they'd grown more dependent on each other and on me and on my sisters. Their diets got stranger, but in different ways. Mother gave up trying to cook for Dad, whose weird eating habits fostered my own. So they ate out, a lot. Even then, I gave scant thought to their mortality. Their quality of life seemed good. Naturally, I counted on them, implicitly and explicitly, to show me how to age with dignity. Wasn't that their job? I saw aging as an extension of their parental responsibility.

I was still in my late thirties when I got the phone call about Dad's lung cancer. While I took care of the elderly at work, and I'd had plenty of deaths in the operating room or during codes and traumas and open heart procedures, my own personal experience with illness was limited. My brain aneurysm was still several years away. Ruthann had had encephalitis as a child, which was terrifying, but she'd recovered. I'd torn up my knee on the ski slopes, and broken a bone or six, but I'd been lucky. Despite the many discussions my dad had forced on us about his own ultimate demise, they had really focused on another aspect of old age: the part you could control. They focused on the finances, the logistics, the less abstract details. *Have a will,* he insisted, *as soon as you have children or any assets. You want to avoid probate. Put your assets in trust. Plan for old age, plan for retirement. Control what you can. Buy term insurance, not whole life, if you have kids and any debt. I do not want to be institutionalized,* he said. *No nursing homes. No long-term hospitalization. No feeding tubes, no ventilators.* He wanted to die at home, surrounded by loved ones. We left it there. As it turns out, that's actually a lot. That's a hell of a lot more than most people do.

Medical school teaches you to think in statistics, like cure rates and life expectancies, and you place your hope in the numbers, that you or your family member will be in that seventy percent that makes it five years, or whatever percentage that responds to chemo. Because that's most people, right? Aren't we most people? Numbers and statistics are just that. When you apply them to someone you love, a skewing takes place, affected by emotion and hope. All along, I had assumed that aging would turn out well for my parents and, by genetic extension, for me too. It's a number fallacy—*a confirmation bias*—that is very hard to let go of. But at some point—and that point was much further down the one way road than it should have been—a different interpretation of those numbers began to take hold. At some lonely moment in the nineteen months my dad had cancer, I realized my loved one might not be in the lucky five or ten or twenty percent that survives beyond two years. I saw the side effects and the complications, and the complications of the side effects. I realized that what begins as straightforward treatment or a simple hospitalization can gradually morph into a multi-week disaster with multi-organ failure not because a loved one isn't getting good care but because a loved one is getting a lot of care. Was it when he had to go back to the operating room for bleeding? The first time, or the second time? When he couldn't pee and had to have his prostate removed? Life gets complicated at the end. I realized that there comes a point in every person's life when less is more. But how do you know when you're at that point? And how do you know it if you don't have the benefit of a physician or a nurse or a healthcare provider in your immediate family, or in the immediate vicinity, having had the luxury of interpreting a *values* discussion with the person who has the disease, who's lying in the hospital bed?

When that call finally came and I heard the words that are inevitable in most adults' lives, I probably could have handled it better than I did. I wish I'd been more compassionate, instead of saying *This should be pretty straightforward*. I knew that life ended. And before it ended, it could slow down to an agonizing speed. I knew this, and some part of me even expected it. I ought to have been prepared because he'd been trying to prepare me for years. But I wasn't ready. I'd been avoiding the conversation he kept having with me, around me, and over me. I'd been happily wearing the lemon juice.

~

Cellular biologists constitute the majority of the country's researchers on aging. That makes sense, I suppose. If you want to understand what drives the body, deconstruct it down to its most fundamental level—the cell. If you can't answer the complicated questions, answer the simplest ones first. There's a connection, complex and difficult to comprehend, between cellular senescence and cancer. It may be that the accumulation of dysfunctional senescent cells disrupts the microenvironment of tissues. Older cells mutate, mutations lead to cancer. The accumulation of mutations might synergize with the accumulation of senescent cells and increase your cancer risk. That seems to be one of the biggest problems, and fears, of aging.

Shortly after publishing his astonishing and important findings regarding the clearing of senescent cells in 2011, Dr. van Deursen lost his NIH grant. Luckily, his lab had other funding.

# Nine

You know the parlor trick,
wrap your arms around your own body
and from the back it looks like
someone is embracing you
her hands grasping your shirt
her fingernails teasing your neck
from the front it is another story
you never looked so alone
your crossed elbows and screwy grin
you could be waiting for a tailor
to fit you with a straight jacket
one that would hold you really tight.

—Billy Collins, 'Embrace'

On a Monday morning in February 1997 I walked the corridors of an excellent community hospital. I was to meet Dad, Mom, and sister Bonnie at 6:30 AM in the pre-surgical area. I felt like an outsider here, but not the average visitor either. I mentally compared my hospital to this one. Better intake rooms here, better traffic flow there. I made mental notes and got lost looking for the Same Day Surgery unit. I found my family in Pre-op where Dad lay on the cart. He wore a hospital gown; a sheet and light blanket covered him. His thick white hair, recently washed, was long and fluffy and smoothed back from his high forehead. His feet hung off the end of the cart. A middle-aged nurse stood by his bedside, chatting with Mom and Bonnie about mutual friends. Dad introduced us. When the nurse left, Dad smiled, shook his head and remarked, "I have no idea who she is. But I can't go anywhere anymore without knowing somebody. *Hello Carl. Long time no see, Carl.* This is what happens when you live too long. You become a goddamn icon. It's ridiculous." He shook his head and I smiled.

My father possessed a wry, dry humor that failed him only under the most difficult of circumstances. I like to think I inherited that resilient humor from him.

"It's nice when people recognize you," Mom scolded. Her humor emerged in calmer settings.

"No, it's not. I hate it. Don't I, honey?" he asked, looking at me.

"Sure, Dad," I said. "Did you get any sleep last night?"

"Of course not. I never get any sleep. I was awake at 4:00 AM."

My mother rolled her eyes. Bonnie said, "If you didn't go to sleep at 8:00, you wouldn't wake up at 4:00. How much sleep does a person need?"

An orderly came to take him to the operating room. A forty-ish man from the Philippines, the orderly introduced himself, then checked my dad's chart and armband to make certain he had the correct person.

"It's nice to meet you, Ben," Dad said. He looked down at his feet sticking out from the end of the cart. "You've probably never seen anyone with such beautiful feet, have you, Ben?"

We all looked down at Dad's feet. They were pronated, perfectly flat, and extremely large. Not that beautiful. His second toe extended a good half-inch beyond his great toe. Those carny feet had kept him out of the military in the Second World War. Dad wore a size 12-1/2 AAAA shoe. Ben cleared his throat. Sometimes I rescued people like Ben, said something conciliatory or attempted to make my family or the situation seem normal or harmless. Sometimes I tried to give some indication that this group—related purely by DNA and circumstance—was simply burdened by a unique brand of humor to which others might not be privy but shouldn't take offense. It's probably a birth order thing: the youngest as diplomat.

But Dad had lung cancer. If he wanted to make jokes, so be it.

"You know, I used to model these feet," Dad said, smiling

and warming to his topic. "In the Sears catalog, back in the sixties. I've always been known for my appendages." He smirked at Mom. "A lot of women wanted me because of these feet."

Mom turned to Ben. "Are you taking him now?"

~

The accident, at the time, seemed so crazy it could have been a joke. A truck ran a red light, broadsiding the local coroner's van, which contained a driver, a front seat passenger, and a stiff in the back. The truck driver died, the van driver died, the passenger nearly died, and the stiff in the back seat stayed dead. The whole thing was so horrific that we made a joke. *The stiff stayed dead.*

~

Years of therapy have taught me to pay as much attention to what I don't remember as to what I do. Which of course isn't easy, given the nature of memory.

Dave, a dear friend and Dad's surgeon, came out to talk to my family after the operation. My sister Erica had arrived also. We sat together in the conference room and Dave described the procedure. I know what these conversations typically consist of; I've heard surgeons give their spiels hundreds of times. But in my father's case, I cannot recall what Dave said about anything, about how much lung he removed, how many lymph nodes he found, whether or not they looked suspicious. I cannot recall a single word. I suppose he found some suspicious lymph nodes, which is why I don't remember.

~

My patient, the front seat passenger, suffered a not unusual combination of injuries: broken pelvis, lacerated spleen, long bone fractures. Because of a prolonged extraction by the EMT's, he had very low blood pressure, very low body temperature, and a very bad prognosis. The emergency department resuscitated him, then brought him to us in the operating room. We did the case in room six, I remember, where the surgeons explored his abdomen, removed his spleen, stabilized the legs, and applied an external fixator to his pelvis, which looked like a giant titanium Tinker toy. For my part, I gave him blood, fluids, drugs, working hard to save him but also biding my time, pretty much, because his blood pressure was fifty to sixty systolic all night long despite vasopressors; I couldn't get it any higher. There was just no way this guy would survive. I mean, we did all we could, but nobody expected him to live. When blood pressure is that low, for that long, one by one the organs shut down—kidney, liver, guts—what's called multi-system failure. Recovery from multi-system failure is highly unusual.

~

A few years before Dad's surgery for lung cancer, he had a bump removed from his neck. The pathology came back as sebaceous cell carcinoma, a rare form of skin cancer that can behave like melanoma, which he'd also had three years prior to that. The doctor said he should have a wider excision of the neck lesion. He refused. My mother called and asked if I'd talk to him. Then the surgeon called me and asked that I plead with him to come back and have the additional surgery. *This thing could spread*, he said, *it could go to his lymph nodes*. I told them both I'd do what I could. I invited my parents over for Sunday dinner.

While I tossed the salad, Dad stood nearby, hands in his pants' pockets, and watched me work. He had a look on his face. Not a good look. It was the kind of look that let me know not to ask for the car or spending money when I was a teenager.

"Dr. Jameson called," I began anyway, "and said he wants you to come back and have more skin taken off of your neck." Dad pursed his lips, cast his eyes down.

"I'm not gonna do it."

I took a deep breath. "Dad, you have to do it," I said. Reasonably, I thought. "You don't have a choice. It's the only way to cure this thing."

He looked up, instantly furious. Ready to shoot the messenger. "I'm not gonna let that guy butcher me. He wants to cut up my neck, do a skin graft." His face went dark pink. "I wouldn't let that goddamn butcher touch me again! If he were the last doctor on earth!"

I felt myself flushing too. Fights with my dad were always like this. His temper flared hot and fast and you'd lost the battle before you realized it had begun. You lost because he was angrier than he had any reason to be. You knew he'd fight dirtier, go for the jugular. "Dad, he just wants to do what's right for you."

"I hate that guy!" he shouted. "My knee has never been right since he operated on me!" The rest of the house went oddly silent around us.

"You've got arthritis. He didn't give you that."

"All I know is I'm not going back, and I won't have anything else done. And you can mind your own goddamn business!"

I looked to Mom, waiting for her to tell him she'd authorized this intervention. She stayed silent, afraid of the monstrous temper he couldn't control. I went upstairs. Dad went home. My husband fed Mom and the kids some dinner, and then drove her home.

I sat alone in my bedroom, dry eyed but sad. My dad wasn't an easy guy, and we'd had our fights over the years, but I felt as though somehow my profession had leveled the playing field between us. It allowed me to hold my own with him, but it didn't allow me to tell him what to do. Where does the doctor end and the daughter begin? We hadn't established our boundaries until that day. He wanted my advice, but then he ignored it; I kept giving it anyway. People are entitled to make their own decisions, even when I think they are wrong. In truth, I didn't know the numbers—no one did. There weren't enough patients with this rare cancer to have good statistics. Parents and children, doctors and patients. The lines were blurry. I had knowledge he didn't have. He had rights I needed to respect. Neither of us apologized or mentioned the argument or the surgery ever again.

~

My van patient was young, big and healthy. The young ones are tough, I used to say, hard to kill. So here's the thing—you just never know. They keep going and going; their hearts don't want to stop. Dying goes against the natural order for those young bodies. You check their blood gases, and the pH is so low, they shouldn't be alive. Normal is 7.4, his was 6.9.

All night long we worked on our patient from the coroner's van, resuscitating him, giving him everything we had; the epinephrine ran full blast. His blood pressure was negligible; he had no urine output for hours. But, surprisingly, he made it through the night...and then the next night...and the next. Later I heard he stroked his spinal cord and his brain because his blood pressure was low for so long. But who thought he'd even make it that far? The neurosurgeons figured he'd be paraplegic and his brain was definitely squash. He'd be a vegetable. Forever impaired. Personally, I thought, I'd rather be dead.

~

Three days after Dad's thoracotomy for lung cancer, I heard masculine voices and laughter coming from his hospital room. I peeked in through the doorway. Harold, his elderly lawyer, occupied the recliner next to Dad. Harold saw me and waved. A young priest with thick glasses and thinning brown hair stood at the foot of the bed, shifting back and forth in Birkenstock sandals worn over white gym socks. A thin, middle-aged man I vaguely recognized sat on a chair in the corner of the small, single room. He appeared tall, but folded up, like a praying mantis.

I stepped past the priest. "Hey Dad." I pressed a kiss to his reddened cheek.

"Hi, honey. Do you know everybody?"

"Sure," I said, and turned. The priest stuck out a hand.

I glanced at the man in the corner. His body seemed wholly asymmetrical, as if gravity came at him from a different angle than it did for you or me. We made eye contact and I said to him, "Melvin, right? We've met at my parents' house." He unfolded upward and stepped toward me, while leaning sideways and backward. Usually people are stoned when they do that.

As I let go of his hand, Melvin winked. I remembered him better, an ectomorphic loner, one of the oddballs that Dad collected. He winked at me again.

After a few minutes, the men cleared out. Dad showed me his rash. It was all over his face, chest and stomach, probably from the antibiotic. I helped him reposition himself in the bed, put some pillows under his knees and fluffed the ones behind his head. A thin tube taped to his back connected him to a medication pump, providing a continuous infusion of narcotics and dilute local anesthetic into the epidural space. He seemed relatively euphoric, a side effect of the medication.

"I've had people here all day," he said, shaking his head as if popularity was an affliction, and he was too busy or important to be sick. "The guys from work brought me papers to sign, we've got a conference call scheduled for tomorrow morning, all day it's been like that. Father Dudley was the third priest to visit today."

"How many times can you take communion in one day?" My remote Catholic training failed me. "Isn't it illegal more than once?"

"You know, I hadn't thought of that," Dad answered. Flushed and puffy with his soft white hair, he looked like a fretful cherub. "I think I had communion three times today. And if Pinky (Dad's neighbor and a Catholic deacon) comes, he'll bring me communion, too. That'd make it four times in one day."

"You'll be very holy," I said.

"Or in big trouble. You can't overdose on that stuff, can you?"

"Eucharist poisoning? I don't think it's been described in the medical literature. Yours could be the first case history. Maybe it's the cause of your rash. Why was Melvin winking at me?"

"Was Melvin winking at you?"

"It was disconcerting."

"I think that's a nervous tic, honey. He winks at me, too." Dad closed his eyes and yawned. Within minutes, he fell asleep.

~

My van patient came back to the operating room several times for urologic and orthopedic procedures. I took care of him again when he had a gastrostomy tube put in; he was too out of it to eat, so nutrition had to be delivered directly to his stomach. But I remember thinking, *this is so sad. So incredibly sad.* Imagine spending the rest of your life strapped into some wheelchair, waiting for people to feed you and wipe spit from your chin. I don't want to live like that. That's everybody's fear, isn't it? That's why it's important to make your wishes known. And this guy was young, maybe four years younger than I. Late twenties. Who thinks about that stuff when you're in your twenties? In the recovery room, the nurses had tied his arms to the side-rails so he couldn't pull any tubes out, which seemed silly; those arms looked completely useless—their muscle definition had faded from fluids and immobility. And even though he smelled bad, like hospital and sweat and old adhesive tape and the sick sweetness of Ensure, there was still something vital about him. As if he was still in there, stuck inside. He was young sick, not old sick, and I could tell that once he'd been handsome and strapping, big and solid and masculine. He looked like somebody who'd play softball in a league after work, then go to a local pub—maybe drink beer, laugh, and play a mean game of foosball. The stiff thing wasn't funny anymore. I forgot why it ever seemed funny in the first place.

~

I relaxed into the recliner beside Dad's hospital bed. It didn't surprise me that he had so many visitors. He was an icon, as he'd said. He reminded me of *The Godfather*, in the way that he listened, and the way that men came to see him for help and guidance. He had a lot of friends, men friends, priests and former priests, married men, single men, from all walks of life. They would come and talk to him. He'd listen and give advice. Having been abandoned by his own father, he believed in being a father figure, for family and non-family alike. He had a way of being fully present for people, of listening intently to their troubles, of never shrinking from conflict or difficult decisions, of being moral but surprisingly nonjudgmental.

~

And then, there were other cases, other traumas, other call nights. I didn't hear anything else about that patient. After four months in the hospital, he transferred to a rehab facility. Then one day the trauma surgeon happened to mention him, told me the guy got better. His spinal cord injury had improved. His brain perked up too. Amazing, he said, like a miracle.

One night I was on call making rounds on the patients scheduled for surgery the next day. It was late, after eleven PM. Most of the patients were asleep already. With the OR schedule in my hands, I ran an eye down the page, made a plan, and went to a ward where I grabbed all the charts I needed, then worked my way down the hall, room to room. I checked the charts, entered the significant anesthesia concerns on our consult sheets, said hi to the patients, and explained what they could expect. After

I'd seen two or three patients on the orthopedics floor, I walked into a single patient room. I glanced at the surgeon's pre-op note: it said orthopedic hardware removal, lower leg.

~

I drove Dad home from the hospital on the sixth post-operative day. He moved cautiously, as his two broken ribs—a by-product of having half a lung removed—were painful. He was quiet on the way home, no jokes, no stories.

My mother waited at the back door. After we settled Dad in his favorite chair in the family room, he told my mother to go upstairs to find him a laxative. His current misery was bowel-related—the drugs had stopped him up. Mom turned to go, but I offered to do it instead.

"There's some suppositories up there, in the cabinet under the sink," Dad told me.

~

The name was Mark something—it didn't seem familiar. Inside the door, the patient had his back to me. He walked carefully, a cane in his right hand, and gently maneuvered himself around and sat on the bed.

"Mr. F.?" I asked. You always have to ask, double-check the names.

"Yes. Mark F." He turned his head and smiled at me. A scar, still healing, dimpled his cheek. Short blond hair barely covered his scalp. His face was clean-shaven and handsome. His smile revealed even white teeth. I blushed a little. Wow, I thought, nice looking man.

"You're here for hardware removal, correct?" I asked, then introduced myself. "I'm from Anesthesia." I explained that I was making pre-operative visits.

"The left leg is the correct leg," he said, as if he'd spent some time in a hospital, knew all about correctly identifying the operative side. He pulled the sheet away to show me where the surgery would be. "They're taking out a plate and three screws." His speech was slow and careful.

"There's not much in this chart," I said, "since you just arrived. Can you tell me the nature of your original injury?"

He smiled again. His hands were limp at his sides. He looked down at them, then smoothed the blanket back over both legs, and folded his hands in his lap. He raised his head; the smile was gone.

"I was a trauma patient. Nine months ago. Broken pelvis, broken legs, ruptured spleen, spinal cord injury." He paused. "But here I am."

I flipped some pages in the chart, searching for helpful clues. Then I checked the name again, and stared hard at him. I remembered checking his name that night, on dozens of bags of blood as I transfused him.

"You were in the coroner's van," I whispered.

"I was."

"I didn't recognize you," I said. A stinging acid settled in my mouth, in the back, near the base of my tongue. "I took care of you twice. That first night, the night of the accident, then again for the G-tube."

"I'm sorry." He shook his head. "I don't remember."

"No," I said. "You wouldn't."

He smiled again and the smile pulled at the scar on his face. "I've been in rehab."

I watched him carefully, blinking hard. "It's amazing. I mean, you're walking and....everything."

"I'm lucky to be alive." His smile faded. For the first time I wondered who might have been in the back of that van. I wondered about the truck driver. And the guy driving the van. They might have been friends.

"Well, you've been through this before," I said, dropping my eyes to the chart, anxious to be gone, not realizing there would be questions I would want to ask. Not about the anesthesia, but for myself, later. Questions about those lost months, how he managed those months. "So you must know the ropes. Nothing to eat or drink after midnight. You need anything? Like a shot pre-op? Help you relax?"

"No thanks." He watched me closely. "Will it be you, tomorrow?"

I shifted the charts in my arms. "No," I said. "I go home in the morning. They let me go home. Anyway, I'm really glad to see how well you're doing. It's incredible. Good luck tomorrow." I backed toward the door, but didn't take my eyes off him until the last second. I heard him say thanks as I turned.

~

I found the package of suppositories after minimal searching. The cabinet beneath Dad's sink fascinated me; it was like a time capsule, circa 1960. A cracked and petrified red rubber hose curled around a mineral-encrusted Water Pik in the back of the cabinet. Beside the Gentian Violet that he used to paint his gums, and the Selsun Blue with which he washed his hair, sat a glass device that resembled a Dachshund without head or legs that he used to snort warm salt water and clean out his sinuses. I used to hide it whenever I had a cold, so my parents weren't tempted to use it on me. I carried the suppositories downstairs.

He had moved to the sofa. "You find them?"

"I found them. Unfortunately, they expired in 1975. At the expected exponential rate of decay, you'd have to stick five of these up your ass to do any good."

"Smart aleck," he smiled and clutched his chest. "Don't make me laugh."

The pupils of his pale gray eyes were small—a side effect, like the constipation, of the narcotics. "You know," he said, "they think I'm cured. Did they tell you that? That I'm cured?"

"Yes, Dad," I said. "That's great news."

He nodded. "That woman doctor, the oncologist, told me she didn't think I'd even need chemo."

I just nodded.

"Stop for some ice cream on the way home from the drug store, wouldja, honey?" He closed his eyes again. His face was still pink from the rash. "Vanilla would be fine."

~

I backed into the hall, bumped into a nursing aide, then excused myself. Still holding the charts, I leaned against the wall outside Mark F's room and closed my eyes. The sting in my throat subsided. I swallowed a few times. After a moment, I stood straight. Not perfect, but composed.

The hardest thing—when I was young—about practicing medicine was learning to balance compassion with dispassion. It was learning to find the right distance, invoke the proper boundaries. It was learning to adopt the proper degree of anesthesia. And then once I found it, I had to let it go.

Someone asked me recently if I believe in miracles. I do, I answered. But I don't depend on them.

# PART THREE

# Ten

The second module of *Managing Healthcare Delivery* began on February 27, 2011, five months after my mother's death. Once again, the Executive Education division of Harvard Business School had given us an extensive amount of preparatory reading. But this time the material didn't interest me much and I found it hard to read through the assigned case studies. The second session had been titled: *Perform*. This referred to the day-to-day management of an organization and we would get into the nitty-gritty of finances, service excellence, decision-making, handling difficult personalities, negotiation, and so on. I knew I excelled at dealing with difficult personalities; after twenty-some years working with surgeons, I could manage Attila the Hun if necessary. Actually I *had* worked with Attila—he was a middle-aged orthopedic surgeon who specialized in joints. But regardless, the assignments were diverse; some proved more interesting than others, many were downright tedious. We were to read *Barbarians at the Gate: The Fall of RJR Nabisco* by Burrough and Helyar. I found the story compelling even though the authors painted a picture of clear disaster from page one. Although it was nonfiction, character drove the plot. But most troubling for me was that we were to read an accounting textbook and pass an exam before we arrived on campus. The textbook sat on my desk gathering dust for over a month before I tried to dig in. I skulked through three chapters, then gave up and opted for the online tutorial.

~

According to Daniel Kahneman, the psychologist who won a Nobel Prize in Economics, people who face a difficult question will usually try—without even realizing it—to answer a simpler question instead.

~

Winters in Chicago should provide the ideal environment to learn accounting. Ice, sleet, and snow limit your more interesting options, so it ought to be comparatively easy to stay inside and ponder which side of the T bar to place a credit or a debit. After a week or so, I came to understand that wherever I thought a credit should go, I was mistaken. And if I deemed something a credit, it turned out to be a debit. I then tried doing the opposite of what I deduced and realized I was still wrong. I couldn't guess, second guess, or third guess myself and come up with the correct answer. Accounting bested me on the mitochondrial level. *I'd been an Illinois State Math Scholar! I'd slept with math textbooks for years—and I'm not being metaphorical!* The situation reminded me of something a resident told me back in medical school: if a med student has a fifty-fifty chance of getting a question right, he (or she) will get it wrong eighty percent of the time. With that in mind, I attacked the basic principles again, knowing that a blindfolded baboon could probably do better. I sighed and engaged in excessive handwringing; I eventually managed to get the basic principles correct. But as soon as the accounting went from simplistic to the slightest bit complicated, I got lost. I flunked the exam. I patiently reviewed the tutorial, and flunked it again. I am not someone accustomed to flunking. It sat poorly upon my ego. We had been given a point person in Cambridge to call with questions; Jeffrey, a PhD candidate in Economics, hinted that I was the only person who had actually contacted him. Jeffrey and I spent hours on the phone together and, despite the fact that he was an excellent teacher and he tried to help and I really tried to understand, accounting didn't happen for me. I developed a mental block around that stupid T-bar. I remembered when I was in high school, frustrated with calculus, and my dad told me to think of it as its own form of logic. As its own language. That helped. I knew that learning accounting probably required a similar leap of faith, intellectually, but I truly didn't give a shit. It also occurred to me that perhaps, like my mom and my grandmother, I might have dementia. Sure it was mild at that point since I was only fifty-two, but I worried anyway. After a lifetime of being strong in math, I could not learn this basic financial information. I worried that if accounting slipped into my brain, something much more important might slip out; I had only so much functional space. I had some pretty important skills I didn't want to lose. What were they again? The threat of dementia loomed huge in my mind, and the threat itself grew by self-perpetuation. I forgot things, therefore I felt certain I had a cognitive disorder. My cognitive disorder affected my ability to communicate. I had trouble finding words. My difficulty with word finding caused me stress. The stress made me forget. And on it went. The endless winter—or what we refer to in Chicago as *seasonal affective disorder*—made everything worse. Mom was gone; my life lacked structure. And my dog, Olga, developed dementia too. She seemed very confused some days. Nobody in my house was going to pass the accounting final.

~

Kahneman explains in his book *Thinking, Fast and Slow* that a commonplace cognitive error is to believe that what you see is all there is. WYSIATI, for short. But what we see is usually only the surface. This is true for people whom we judge based on appearances or gestures or emails or promises, and it is true for situations about which we know a smattering of facts. What we hear is only a fraction of what has happened. People are so much more and, often, so much less than we expect. As my friend Dave used to say, never assume. If I were to learn accounting, maybe I could push it into the part of my brain that assumes, and push the assuming part out.

~

I sought help from my therapist.

"I can't pass the accounting final," I said. I sat in the same chair every time. I didn't go for the sofa. God only knows what might have come out of me if I'd lain down on that sofa. "There's something wrong with me."

"The fact that you can't pass accounting makes you normal." My therapist had the look of a hot nerd about him, like Albert Einstein after a day at Elizabeth Arden.

"You're not helping."

"What do you want me to say? I couldn't pass accounting either. Especially not now." So the similarity to Einstein didn't extend beyond the physical. "Those brain cells are long gone. And good riddance."

"What is it about math? It's like I've traded in some part of my brain for something else. But what? And why does it have to be that way? My math brain has ceased to function. I'm all gooey and distracted."

"What do you think it means?"

"Do you think it means I have dementia?" I asked. I know he thought I was kidding, but I wasn't.

"No, I think it means that you're stressed. And stress can affect your memory. As can grief. You have lots of reasons not to want to learn accounting, Margaret. I'd say that number one is that you're not interested. Do you really need accounting at this point in your life? And I think you're still grieving."

He was right as usual. I did not want to learn accounting. And I couldn't get a handle on my grief. I didn't feel entitled to it because my mom had been really old and had dementia and had been suffering. It was her time and now she was no longer suffering and, for those reasons, I shouldn't feel lost and lonely without her. So instead of missing her I should have been glad she was gone. But instead I missed her so much I could barely breathe. Her life had given meaning and structure to mine for years. It had given me an excuse not to have a life. And even though she hadn't been able to communicate because of her dementia, I still felt the person she used to be, and that's the person I missed and grieved for. What the hell was grief, anyway?

In the winter after Mom died, I came to depend on my dog for almost everything—companionship, advice, more companionship. But even my dog seemed to be channeling my mother, or at least her senility.

My poor, sweet, elegant mutt, Olga, stood in front of the mirror in our hallway and stared at herself as if to say, *Who the heck is that?* At night, as she fell asleep she would dig and dig, creating havoc on my carpeting. She had trouble getting up and lying down. Her hips obviously ached; she couldn't tolerate the pain medicine the vet had prescribed, and her stomach grew more fragile every day. She puked everywhere. Her bowels defined unpredictable. Luckily I have a leopard print wool carpet so the stains blend in and it tolerates frequent washing. I cooked homemade meals for her, poached chicken thighs, added rice with some broth, a little pumpkin for fiber. I slipped an antibiotic powder in to help regulate the bacteria in her gastrointestinal tract. I should have tried that on my mom when she was alive, to help her bowels. Then, one day, Olga simply stopped eating the chicken and rice. *Enough is enough.* I happened to be eating a hamburger for dinner. I gave her some of that. She liked it. So then she had hamburger *with a bun* every day for breakfast and dinner. At lunch I gave her some high protein prescription dog food with a little beef and bun thrown on top. It didn't fool her. She hated the dog food. She might have been demented, but she knew what she liked.

As I prepared for the second Harvard Business School session, I realized it was like a massively condensed version of an MBA program: how to run an organization as if your life depended on it. Only my life didn't depend on it. In another place, perhaps another time, I might have cared, might have wanted to run something. But that time had passed for me. I had to face facts. Running a business, or a hospital, or any organization—medical or otherwise—didn't seem like something that my future held. I wish it did. I think I might have enjoyed business. The course organizers had set aside considerable time to discuss options for our final project, which would involve developing a business plan. *A business plan…for what?*

I arrived in Cambridge on a grim winter Sunday and once again Dr. Bohmer gave a dynamic lecture on the dire outlook for our current healthcare system. He summarized the course for the next week. Learn the essentials of finance, financial management. Learn about controlling costs, personnel, performance, and negotiation. Maybe I would finally understand the accounting concepts that had eluded me. I promised myself I would attend every extra lecture, every extra help session on finance. Because I would be a good student until I dropped dead, with or without dementia. The week would include presentations given by attendees from different countries where healthcare costs were controlled: the National Health Service in the UK, the Australian system, and Singapore. But I kept coming back to a few concepts that had interested me all along. How do you make a difference, even just a small difference? How do you alter one little thing that will evolve into a ripple effect? Can you effect really meaningful change, even minor change, related to healthcare legislation, by tinkering with the supply side of things? Doesn't true transformation arise from a revolution in demand? Or perhaps from revolution itself?

During one of his lectures, Dr. Bohmer made an interesting statement: "There is no good way to pay physicians."

He went on to compare the strengths and weaknesses of various systems, such as fee-for-service, employment models, pay-for-performance, value-based-purchasing (bundled payments), and accountable care organizations. He briefly touched on the coming changes in fee structures, but his core argument—that physicians must be incentivized to work just like every other person on the planet—seems like a tenet that no one wants to touch. Fee-for-service gets the most work and the most innovation out of the most talented individuals. And we have a system that can't afford the expense but doesn't want to give up the innovation, the productivity, or lose the talent. We have an inflated sense of how great American medicine is that seemingly justifies the runaway costs. But the fact remains that other countries manage to provide excellent care for less money, and with far less aggravation.[xi,xii] Perhaps their guiding principles are different from ours. Perhaps this is an understatement.

As I sat through lecture after lecture, it occurred to me that healthcare reform requires a group think mentality. But we are not a group think country.

We have become defined, even imperiled, by special interests. Healthcare as a percentage of gross domestic product is fifty percent higher in the United States than in any other developed country, and Americans have a shorter life expectancy. [xiii] It seems safe to say that healthcare has been *bankrupting us* while simultaneously denying adequate care to tens of millions of Americans for years. Why is that? Well, that requires a complicated answer beyond the scope of this book. But as Kahneman suggests, people who cannot answer a complex question will answer a simpler one instead.

Medicine is not a business as we think of other typical, revenue-generating industries. I can choose whether I want to buy a car, a new car, a used car, what brand, the kind of mileage it gets, and so forth. I can choose the timing of my purchase and how I will pay it off. But if I get breast cancer, I have to take care of it right now, someplace near my home because I will have to continue working as much as I can and try to somehow manage to have the treatment I need while getting to and from my job. Will I even be able to keep my job? I will be frightened, not just for my own health, but for my kids and what it means for them in the short term and the long term, about the potential surgery and chemotherapy and radiation, and the recovery. And what if I have any number of possible complications? What if the nodes are positive? What if my income drops significantly? Will I need to sell my home? Will I be able to continue living and working as I have been? Will I need to change my lifestyle? Will my life ever be normal again? You don't consider the same issues when you weigh a Hyundai versus a Ford, because purchasing a car does not cause nausea and vomiting, hair loss, or potential bankruptcy.

Somehow, buying treatment for breast cancer just doesn't fit into the same business model as buying a car. But we—as a nation—pretend that it does, because some people have excellent insurance to offset the cost. Some people have better resources all around. We pretend the emotional ramifications of health issues don't come to bear on healthcare as an industry. But I think they're inseparable. I think that healthcare as an industry, as well as the members of Congress, don't know what they don't know. Which is why healthcare thinks it's in the car business. We legally sanction for-profit hospitals because, if there's money to be made, if we subject pain and suffering to the competitive marketplace, things usually improve, right? But I find the concept of for-profit hospitals appalling. There's an inherent misalignment of motives in the "business" of medicine. Physicians and hospitals have a *moral and financial incentive* to provide excessive care to people who can pay for it as long as they have a heartbeat. Hospitals don't have morals, but are guided by balance sheets, boards, and public opinion. CEO's are driven by revenue and strategic career moves. The intrinsic quandaries are innumerable. People, including children, get hurt, develop diseases for which they require complex therapies; hurt people don't get taken care of because they lack insurance, education, or any of a whole host of resources. Or they are taken care of in the acute phase because emergency rooms cannot turn them away: but then they are lost to follow-up. Specialties operate in silos; coordination of care is mostly a joke. All of this—each and every person without adequate healthcare regardless of the newly implemented and embattled ACA—has a profound effect on the economy, not only on the cost to our system, but on the long-term productivity of our entire population. That is a piece of this puzzle no one wants to address because it's not quantifiable, except to manipulate and push the agenda of one political party over another. Both are guilty. And when the profit motive cannot be removed from the pretext of *medical necessity*, as is the case far more often than the public realizes—a perfect example is the medical robotics industry—there is something radically wrong.

Medical care has risks, expensive risks, many of which are never explained in adequate detail, probably because some patients would opt out. Patients—for their part—rarely perform adequate due diligence on their own diseases and treatments. They don't take responsibility for their health. It isn't within my control whether I get a brain aneurysm and spend the rest of my life with migraine headaches. It isn't within your control whether you have a family history of heart disease. What is within our control is acquiring knowledge about our diseases, our general state of health, and our response to that knowledge. That's where way too many people wear the lemon juice.

~

Cognitive errors abound in the rhetoric surrounding healthcare reform. If you want to take a lesson from the medical malpractice literature, read up on the *framing effect*, the *fundamental attribution error*, the *outcome bias*, the *overconfidence bias*, the *premature closure bias*, the *sunk costs bias*, the *unpacking principle*, *vertical line failure*, and the *visceral bias*, to name but a few. All of these demonstrate ways in which our thinking and decision-making about an individual's medical care can be screwed up. But the same principles apply broadly to the way we frame the delivery of medical care—we're just too close to see it. In their seminal paper entitled "Judgment under Uncertainty" published in *Science* in 1974, Amos Tverskey and Daniel Kahneman state: "What is perhaps surprising is the failure of people to infer from lifelong experience such fundamental statistical rules as regression toward the mean, or the effect of sample size on sampling variability."[xiv] In the paper, they address the heuristic that describes the probability of an event under uncertainty. In other words, people fail to learn from experience, from basic principles of math, from basic principles of chance. They make decisions based on poor instincts and bad judgment. This helps to explain our nation's health care policy.

~

I kept going back to statistics published by the Centers for Medicare and Medicaid Services: Medicare costs in the last year of life represented a disproportionate amount of the total—consistently in excess of twenty-five percent over the past twenty years. Polls repeatedly find that seventy percent of Americans want to die at home while the data show that seventy percent of Americans actually die in hospitals. So Americans are not getting the care they want. Canadians feel similarly about end-of-life care, with approximately seventy percent dying in hospital. Only the Canadian system allows them to identify the variance as a problem, study it, and look at ways to improve the delivery of care. But that doesn't happen in any organized fashion here. Why is that? Could it be that there's a profit motive to keep people in the hospital? Could it be that we perform procedures on the dying, causing more pain and suffering, under the guise of prolonging life? That's how hospitals make money. Patients do not die sooner in hospice; if anything, they seem to live longer[xv]. And the cost of death in hospice is about a third of the cost of an in-hospital death; but we're not supposed to talk about that. Talking about cost is taboo, as if taking the cheaper option automatically means you're getting substandard care. But here's the rub: it isn't true. Powerful emotional and cultural factors contribute to poor communication and a lack of planning by patients. There is also a documented unwillingness by physicians to address end-of-life issues with patients, and a well-established financial incentive to keep them hospitalized. These factors together conspire to keep patients in the hospital where they experience a more prolonged, institutional, invasive, and less satisfying death. There are all sorts of rational reasons for end-of-life to be managed better—more humanely and ultimately more cost-effectively—than we are doing now. We know how to do it. But the incentives aren't aligned. *How do we shift this paradigm?*

I thought back to some of the codes I had attended over my professional lifetime. By law, everyone who dies in the hospital must be resuscitated unless there is a Do Not Resuscitate order on the patient's chart. A fraction of hospitalized patients have that order on their charts for a whole variety of reasons. For some it makes perfect sense to attempt resuscitation, but for many, particularly the ones who are most likely to die, or "arrest", it does not make any sense at all. The people most likely to be resuscitated are the people who die unexpectedly. Elderly patients with cancer, patients with multi-organ failure, patients with end stage heart or lung disease who have had multiple hospitalizations, truly sick people—these are often the patients who rarely survive resuscitation to discharge.

I finished my week in Boston. I still didn't understand accounting, but I learned the basics of writing a business plan. It wasn't that different from writing a book proposal. I just had to come up with an idea that utilized my skills and my knowledge; there was no shortage of problems to be solved.

# Eleven

It didn't show itself immediately, but within six months of his surgery, Dad's cancer came back. He never fully recovered from the thoracotomy, never gained back the weight he'd lost. The disease, when it recurred, settled in his liver, pushing aside his stomach and distending his abdomen. It irritated his diaphragm. He had chronic hiccups, belched constantly, and complained of a persistent burning pain that sat in the middle of his chest.

The first oncologist he saw suggested no treatment. Dad said he wasn't ready to die, then found another doctor. He had his first chemotherapy in November 1997. A few days later, I drove to my parents' house after work and let myself in the back door.

Mom stood in the kitchen, getting dishes out of the cupboard.

"I'm going to make him Jell-O," she told me before I closed the door. "He likes Jell-O." She looked up at me. Fear widened her eyes. She looked older than I'd ever seen her. "He hardly ate any lunch."

"Forget about meals," I said. "Give him liquids. As much as you can get down him. Chicken broth, Ensure, nothing acidic. No orange juice or pop. Avoid bubbles. If his esophagus is sore, bubbles won't help."

"Hi, honey," he called weakly from the family room.

He sat in a blue upholstered lounge chair with his eyes closed, swollen feet resting on the ground in red plaid slippers. A thin cotton blanket lay draped across his lap. His white hair stuck out in tufts. I kissed his cool cheek then sat down across from him. His breathing was shallow, interrupted frequently by hiccups.

Mom had followed me into the family room. "Do you want some Jell-O?" she asked, standing uncertainly before him.

"Maybe some cantaloupe," he answered.

"Why don't you have some nice cherry Jell-O?"

"Because I want cantaloupe," he said.

Mom straightened her shoulders and turned back to the kitchen. He called, "I'll have Jell-O later."

"How're you feeling?" I asked him.

"Not so good. I have a lot of discomfort here." He pointed to the middle of his chest. "Do you think there's something wrong with me? Could it be my heart?"

"I think your esophagus is sore from the chemo, and your stomach is pushed to the side by the liver. Those two things together make it hard to get stuff down. You should stick to liquids."

Mom came back with a small white ceramic bowl containing a few pieces of cantaloupe.

"Thanks, honey," he said. "Just set them here, on this table. I don't have much of an appetite."

"Did the doctor give you anything for that pain in your esophagus?" I asked.

"I don't know," he said. "I've got so many bottles, I don't know what any of them are for. Lyd, do we have any Tylenol?"

"Would you like a Tylenol?" Mom echoed.

"Yeah, I think maybe I would."

"Did they give you anything for pain, Dad? Something stronger than Tylenol?" I asked.

"Oh, he doesn't like to take that stuff," Mom answered. "It knocks him out so."

"Why don't I look at all the drugs you've got here before I go home, okay?" I said. "Maybe make a chart for you, of what to take for what problem."

"That would help," Mom said. "They give you so much stuff, and when I call the office to ask questions, they're either closed, or they say they'll call me back, and then they don't. It's very frustrating."

"That doctor," Dad said, "the woman oncology doctor, she said I wouldn't suffer." He looked over at Mom. Something passed silently between them. "Didn't she, Lydia? She said they'll give me medicine and I won't ever suffer."

I sat until he fell asleep. I didn't want to think about him suffering. I didn't want to think about the ways physicians throw words around, placating patients and families, soothing themselves. Patients hang onto those words long after their expiration date. And doctors don't like to give patients bad news. I believe it is so difficult, that when they finally deliver it, they make it sound like something it isn't. Like good news, or not-so-bad news. They present it in a way that leaves it open to interpretation.

I glanced at Dad's calm, dozing face. In sleep he would find anesthesia and respite, but a price would be paid, a decremental loss of moments, and the moments between moments, of all that remained. I couldn't help but think about time. There's an eternity in each hour for people going through chemo. You hear it in their voices, especially if you talk to them more than once a day.

Hope, particularly in the setting of cancer, remains a fraught and complex issue. We believe that patients need hope. Perhaps they do. We certainly try to avoid the alternative, which is fear, or acceptance, I suppose. But often we ask patients to hope that what is obvious, straightforward, and standing directly in front of them, facing them in the mirror each day, is not actually so. We prefer they believe in the lemon juice. And a lot of doctors are happy to supply it—in fact they make a living that way. That's the world of medicine as we know it. We pretend that we—physicians—know best. And patients often believe us. Because we're all they've got. But much of the time all we really know is how to prolong suffering. Maybe that's all there is.

While Dad napped, I sat at the kitchen table with a copy of the Physician's Desk Reference. Mom put on her reading glasses, then brought me bottle after bottle of pills, liquid medications, mouthwashes, and salves. She brought me the instruction sheets from the oncologist's office, which listed about half of the medications he was actually given. Sometimes medications are prescribed for their lesser effects rather than for their most common usages. So the label of the drug they'd given Dad for hiccups actually said the medicine was for nausea. Dad didn't have nausea, so he didn't take anything, just continued to hiccup but then couldn't sleep. The drug they prescribed for hiccups at night made him confused but not sleepy, and Mom occasionally found him wandering around the kitchen at three in the morning, looking for his wallet. That scared her, so then she didn't get much sleep, getting up to check on him several times during the night. I noticed there were several different medications, of varying efficacy, for treatment of the same symptoms, but no indication of what should be taken first, or in what order of expected effectiveness. I made a chart, listing drugs Dad should take every day, then drugs he might take if needed, with lists of indications and side effects. My mother studied it, and then taped it to the kitchen wall, above the microwave where all the medications sat together in a shoebox.

After Dad's nap, he felt better. We talked about work, both his and mine.

After a lull, I said, "I think I need a new career."

"And do what?"

"I dunno. What do you think about landscape architecture?"

"I don't think about it. What's the problem?

"I'm not sure I'm cut out for this."

"For medicine?"

"I guess." We were quiet for a while. I was a kid when I made the decision to go to medical school. What did I know at seventeen? I was learning, slowly, that perhaps medicine wasn't the problem; it was having a dad with cancer. But I couldn't tell him that. I could barely think it. *The patient is the one with the disease.*[xvi] You go crazy if you think too much about the suffering. On the other, if you don't think about it, you turn into one of those doctors who lies.

"Would you go back to school?"

"I don't know. Maybe."

"Well, that's something to think about."

"Yeah, it is."

"So what about you?" I asked.

"What do you mean?"

I didn't know what to say, other than the obvious, and I couldn't bring myself to do it. If Dad didn't want to talk about dying, I had to respect his wishes. After all, he'd been talking about it his whole life.

On my way out the door, Mom put her hand on my arm.

"Thanks for coming, honey," she said, and we hugged. "You cheer him up. I can't always do that."


By early February, Dad had undergone two more rounds of chemotherapy, and his tumor was definitely responding. His abdomen had shrunk, the hiccups were gone, and he was eating again. The oncologist gave her the okay for a trip to Florida. So they packed up and went.

Near the end of March, Mom called from Boca Raton.

"Margaret, I'm fine, except for a little problem I'm having with my breathing," she said, "and a tight feeling across my chest and up into my neck. I had it before, back when Dad got sick, but now I get it all the time, even when I'm not doing anything."

Oh boy.

Before I could respond, Mom added, "Oh, and I'm getting these extra beats all the time. I can't even make up the bed without getting dizzy. Do you think I need more exercise?"

My mother was a thousand miles away, on the verge of a heart attack, and she wanted to exercise.

"Mom, I wouldn't exercise just now. Right now actually I'd just sit down. Don't go anywhere. Okay?"

"What's wrong?" she asked. "You're making me nervous."

"Don't worry about a thing, Mom." *Shit, shit, shit.* I'm going to give her a heart attack. "Uh, take an aspirin."

Back in December, in the middle of Dad's second round of

chemo, she'd flunked her stress test and told the doctor she had more pressing things to do than have a cardiac evaluation. Then they went to Florida. And I—her daughter the doctor—*forgot about it.*

My sandals clapped loud against the polished hospital floor, echoing down the long, empty corridor. In the dark waiting room, I called the nurses' station in the Cardio Vascular Intensive Care Unit, identifying myself as Lydia's daughter. A nurse said to come right back. I'd arrived at 6:00 AM, when the nursing staff would be tired but forthright after a twelve-hour shift.

Nancy, a curly-headed nurse with a hundred years of experience, placed a hand on my arm. "I just want to warn you, your mom's a little confused," she said. Okay. It surprises me that more patients aren't confused after bypass surgery. The pump run (cardiopulmonary bypass machine that allows the heart to stop so that surgery can be performed), the sleep deprivation (normal REM sleep is interrupted in ICU's), advanced age, unfamiliar surroundings, and narcotics add up to confusion. So I was prepared.

But the mesh vest on top of Mom's hospital gown indicated more than a little confusion. Sashes attached the vest, and my mother, to the hospital bed.

"She kept trying to get out of bed during the night," Nancy volunteered. "We finally thought it best to put the Posey restraints on her."

"Hey, Mom." I bent over to kiss her cheek. Blood stained the sheet beside her left arm. I glanced at Nancy.

"She took her IV out a while ago. We had to put another one in." She turned to Mom and spoke in a loud voice, "Lydia, you know you have to keep that IV in your arm for a few more days. So don't take it out, okay?"

Mom watched Nancy, then looked at me, disgust on her face. "They won't let me off this cruise ship. I keep telling them I want to go home. These people are good for nothing. And they keep feeding me green Jell-O."

"Lydia, I told you a minute ago that I ordered you some nice red Jell-O. It should be here any minute." Nancy lowered her voice. "She's a little fidgety," she whispered. "And a little cranky, too. She needs a nice long nap."

Nice Jell-O. Nice nap. Mom always said, "Eat your nice beans, dear." She was getting it back in spades.

"They have the worst food here," Mom said. "I don't understand how this cruise line stays in business."

"Mom," I sat down beside her, took her hand in mine, "do you know who I am?"

"Of course I do. Don't you know who you are? Call your father for me, I want to go home. I feel seasick."

"How's your chest feel?" I asked. "Are you having any pain?"

"Oh, a little."

"Mom, do you remember having heart surgery?"

"I forgot. That's tomorrow, isn't it?"

"No," I said, "it was two days ago. You're all done. Everything went very well. Now you just have to get strong again."

"I thought this was a cruise ship."

"It's Intensive Care." Which is similar to a cruise ship, insofar as people throw up a lot, it's expensive, boring, and awful meals are included. And when you're there, you'd rather be anywhere else.

# Twelve

In the early fall of 1998, when Dad was dying, I tried to grapple with my complicated feelings for a complicated man who had been wonderful and awful and done the best job he could. On a September afternoon, I sat alone on the screened porch and gazed at my garden. Once I knew the names of the perennials, the trees, and the grasses. I used to grow plants from seeds in the basement, in elaborate tiered tables with suspended growing lights, and then relocate the plants to the yard. I had more energy then. One year, when my daughters were little, I grew four hundred petunias in the basement, then transplanted them all into an annual border along the side of the house. I don't think I pinched them back properly; they grew very spindly. Since then I'd moved to a different house and begun paying someone to take care of the yard. He wore bulging muscles, cowboy boots, short shorts, and a cowboy hat while working. Suburban lawn care obviously requires a competitive business strategy. The telephone rang.

My mother's voice sounded far away.

"Your father went to the doctor today. That pain he's been having in his shoulder is a growth. The bone scan showed a couple of spots. They're going to give him radiation."

"Where?" I asked. When cancer metastasizes to bones, it eats away at the sensitive periosteum and the pain can be hard to control.

"His hip and his arm. The radiation doctor wants him to see an orthopedic surgeon first; he thinks the arm might break. They said he couldn't play golf or go swimming. And he needs to be careful just getting out of a chair."

"Does the spot on the hip hurt?" If it didn't yet, it probably would soon.

"No. But the shoulder is giving him terrible problems. He's really uncomfortable. He hardly uses the arm anymore."

"Well, the radiation should help the pain."

"They said it won't cure his cancer."

"No. But it should stabilize the bone. It should help the pain."

"So this won't cure him?"

"No."

And it might not help the pain, either.

At the orthopedic surgeon's office, Dad moved slowly, his right arm supporting his left arm beneath the elbow. He kept it tucked against his waist, careful not to bump it. I sat between him and Mom in the waiting room. Mom put on her glasses and picked up a pamphlet about hip replacements. Dad stretched his legs out, crossed them at the ankles, and stared straight ahead. I took a book out of my purse, but didn't read it.

"I don't want to live like this," he said to me, quietly, so my mother couldn't hear. "If this is all I can do, I don't want to live."

"Let's wait and see what the doctor says." I glanced over at Mom. Sometimes I was grateful for her deafness.

After two weeks of radiation, Dad's arm pain hadn't improved. If anything, it had worsened. He took narcotics round the clock. He couldn't drive. We waited about fifteen minutes until his name was called, then all three of us went back to an exam room. An X-ray technician took Dad away for a few minutes for a film of his proximal humerus, where a tumor was lodged. A little while later, Dr. Jim O'Connor came in with a copy of the X-ray.

He perched a hip on the small desk of the exam room. A thin, wiry haired, middle-aged Irishman, he shook Dad's hand, then Mom's, then mine. He and I already knew each other—our kids went to school together. He told Dad to call him Jim, and said that his parents knew them from the golf club. He asked Dad for his medical history, then showed us the X-ray. He pointed out normal bone, where cancer had invaded the humerus, and discussed the risks inherent in leaving the arm untreated.

"So, this is a long, complicated way of saying I think you

need to have the arm stabilized. We do this surgically by making a small incision on the top of the shoulder, the placing a steel rod in through the head of the humerus, down through the middle of the bone. The procedure takes about 45 minutes, you'd need to stay overnight, but you could go home the next day."

"Would there be a lot of pain?" Dad asked.

"Some, but not terrible. We'll give you pain medications. I can't tell you the pain you have currently will disappear immediately, but within a few weeks, the arm should start to feel significantly better."

"Will I be able to swim again? Or play golf?"

"Yes, I would think so. Now, it may be six weeks or so, but I'd say you should be able to do those things again."

Jim turned away to make notes on the chart. In the moment of quiet, Mom cleared her throat, then asked, "So it won't get better on its own?"

"That's not likely. And if the arm fractures, it can be very difficult to stabilize it, and hard to manage the pain. The sooner we do this, the better off Carl will be."

"I see," she said. She and Dad looked at each other then, and she reached out to grip his good hand. Dad nodded at her, glanced briefly at Jim, then looked back down at the floor. Jim told us to plan on surgery the next Tuesday, explained the details of the hospital routine, shook our hands, and then left the room. Mom helped Dad put his jacket on. We walked to their car and they got in.

I pulled the safety belt out and across Dad, gave the buckle to Mom. She snapped it in, then we said good-bye.

I looked for my car in the parking lot, turning slowly, trying to remember where I'd left it. The temperature had dropped and the wind was picking up, clouds darkened the western sky. It would probably rain tonight, I thought, and then shivered, though it was still warm. I saw my car in the far corner of the lot. I didn't remember parking it there.

After one more round of chemotherapy, Dad's oncologist told him she wouldn't give him any more; it wasn't working. She said she had nothing left to offer him. Tumor filled his liver and displaced his stomach; hiccups came and went, staying days at a time. It was hard for him to eat, painful to swallow, and he suffered from constant belching and nausea. The feeling of fullness in his chest had returned. His arm pain was better, but he took oral morphine twice a day, and the arm remained useless. The radiation treatment to his hip had not helped; he'd developed pain there too. The orthopedic surgeon was afraid Dad's hip would fracture just from the simple act of getting out of a chair.

"How long do I have to live?" Dad asked the oncologist.

"It could be three days or three weeks," she said.

He left the office, angry. "What does she know?" he asked no one in particular.

He still went to work every day. One of the guys from the factory came and picked him up. They had installed railings in all the stairwells so that he could use his good arm to go up and down. They'd rented a scooter for him, so that he could motor around the plant, visiting the men who ran the machines. Most of them had worked there for decades. He knew everyone by name; he knew their families, their kids, their stories. They felt comfortable sitting in his office, asking him for advice.

So when he stopped going to work, when he stayed at home wearing pajamas and a bathrobe and let people come to visit him, I knew we were near the end. People called and came from all over the country to say good-bye, including people he'd fired long before, ex-boyfriends and ex-husbands of my sisters. Friends and relatives and former employees came to see him, to visit one last time, people who'd worked with him as well as friends from childhood; they all came to say what they had to say.

"What do we do now?" Mom asked me on the phone. "I don't

mean to keep bothering you, but I don't know who else to call. Last night he had terrible pain in his side. The left side. Terrible pain. I didn't know what to do. I called the doctor's answering service. Nobody called me back. Now this morning, he has a temperature. He hardly eats or drinks anymore. He's so weak, just getting out of the chair is hard."

She was crying. "I'm sorry," she said. "I don't mean to bother you."

"It doesn't bother me. You need to talk about it."

"Last night, at midnight, I couldn't sleep. I went in to his room, you know, to check on him like I do several times during the night. And I lay down beside him and put my arms around him. I didn't want to hurt him. And he cried in my arms." She blew her nose quietly. "I don't know how you do this. How you can work around dying people."

A few days later, I let myself in through the back door at my parents' house. We had contacted hospice, and a nurse appropriately named Grace had come and talked to Dad. He now had a hospital bed in the family room, on the first floor of their house. My sister, Beth, had flown in from Florida. Her kids would be arriving soon. Mom stood at the kitchen sink, rinsing dishes from lunch. Even though she had a dishwasher, she would still wash them by hand. It gave her something to do. She lifted her head, straightened her shoulders, and then looked over at me. I kissed her and she hugged me hard. I glanced into the family room, but nobody was in there.

"Suzy's giving Dad a massage in the living room."

"Can I go in?" I asked.

"Sure. Beth's there too."

I walked through the dining room and front hall. Dad lay face up on a massage table in the living room, covered with a white sheet. I stopped abruptly and raised a hand at the masseuse. Suzy stood on the far side of the portable table, gently massaging his right arm. My dad looked dead. White, cachectic. In profile I barely recognized him. All the flesh was gone from his body. His skin was thin and powdery looking. I glanced down at his chest to check for the movement of breathing. He opened his eyes and they turned towards me.

"I've never had an audience for a massage before. Good thing I'm not naked."

"No kidding."

Beth and I sat in the corner of the living room. When my parents originally bought the house in the fifties, this area was a sun porch. Some years later they enclosed it. Opposite us was my grandmother's Steinway piano, a medium sized grand on which she'd played and given lessons. Per the family lore, Bing Crosby had been a pupil. All four of us girls learned to play; I took lessons until I was eighteen. My dad taught himself late in life. I don't think he ever learned to read music exactly; he just liked to sit and pick out tunes, like the theme song from *Doctor Zhivago* or *Mack the Knife*. Sunlight came in low and angled, yet the room seemed dim. I watched Suzy and thought it can't be easy to massage someone with cancer throughout his bones. That was her special gift.

"Can you fix this pillow under my head, Suzy?" he asked. "It hurts back there."

Beth leaned close to me and whispered, "Why would his head hurt?"

"Mets," I said quietly, though I didn't know for sure. "Bony metastases in his skull."

Our eyes met, then she nodded and looked away. "Grace was here this morning," Beth said, referring to the hospice nurse. "She brought morphine liquid. She's coming back on Monday to show us how to give him subcutaneous injections. For when he can't swallow the pills anymore."

Later that afternoon, Dad lay in the hospital bed in the family room. I sat in the rocker beside him when suddenly he started to talk. He knew I was there, but it didn't seem to matter. He spoke to himself more than to me; I recognized the process as he took inventory, reviewed his life. He was making peace with his past actions or with his inaction; I think he tried to come to terms with his mistakes. I had read about this process. Now I was seeing it in action. It seemed different, though, when it's someone you know, when it's a parent. Reading about it makes it feel like a plot element in a novel. When it happened right in front of me, I thought: *you're leaving out some pretty important stuff, Dad. Where's the apology for being mean, for making me cry all those times, for your sharp tongue, your biting put-downs?* I wanted to hear him purge, but I didn't get to write this script. I realized, not for the first time, it was his life, his death, and his time for reflection. I could only listen, learn, and bear witness.

He talked a little about his regrets. And then he told me a story. I sat and rocked rhythmically looking out the window at the college practice field behind the house where I grew up with the lousy garden and shitty soil. The trees were bare of leaves.

"Vernon came to see me about twenty years ago," Dad said, referring to a guy he'd known for years. Vernon had sought Dad's advice in the past. "He told me he needed to talk. I think we're related somehow, distant cousins or some such. And he said it was important; there was some urgency about it." I thought of *The Godfather* again. Dad was a skinnier version of Vito Corleone, without the hat or raspy voice. And, of course, without the Mafia connections. But over his lifetime, he had played the role of respected advisor for many men from many walks of life. Dad understood moral reasoning as well as moral behavior, and that some people—dangerous individuals—could have the former without the latter. Less sophisticated folk could learn to act morally without understanding why. Dad tried to give advice that encompassed both the moral rationale and the resulting behavior, while also taking practical matters into consideration. He understood that by the time someone came to see him, the easy answers had been exhausted.

I thought he had fallen asleep, but he was just resting. "Vernon told me that his marriage was bad. He said he no longer loved his wife and that he wanted to leave her. You know he was very religious, and so this was a real problem. Religious guys like Vern didn't just leave women they'd been married to for twenty years. He didn't know what to do. He was devoted to his family, but couldn't see himself spending the rest of his life with someone he didn't love."

I said nothing. Now this was some juicy deathbed gossip.

"I didn't think long before giving him my opinion. I told him to stay with his wife. He'd taken a vow; he could work on the marriage and he could find a way to love her again. And so Vernon stayed with his wife."

But as he lay in bed, starving and stripped of all pretense and ego, letting go of everything that protected him from painful self-awareness, letting go of his own protective lemon juice, my dad just shook his head. His beautiful thick white hair was long gone. "You know," he turned to glance out at the gray November day, "I think I made a mistake. I gave him the wrong advice. His wife was an awful person, and I think he would have been happier if he'd left her. He deserved to be happy. We all do." He turned back to me and raised his eyebrows. "Who did I think I was? What right did I have to tell him that?"

By Saturday morning Beth's two daughters had arrived. I drove to my parents' house with my two girls. Dad sat bonelessly at the end of the couch, talking on the phone, a hand covering his face. I saw his shoulders shake and then realized he was crying.

"What's going on?" I asked Beth.

"He's saying his good-byes," she told me. "He's been on the phone all morning." She mentioned the names of close friends and business associates who'd called.

We sat quietly together for several minutes. I wanted to give him privacy, but I didn't want to leave the room. I picked up the newspaper and started reading. Beth wrote out a grocery list. Finally, she put a hand on my arm, and said, "One of us will need to say the eulogy."

I nodded at her and went back to the newspaper. I'd been thinking the same thing.

"What do you want for breakfast?" Mom asked him. "Would you like to try a piece of toast? Or maybe a sliced banana? Or some Ensure with ice cream?" She wrung her hands, trying again to think of something Dad would like to eat.

He looked up at her, fatigue etched into the lines on his face. Beth and I sat at the kitchen table; Bonnie hovered in the kitchen. My sister Erica perched on the edge of the sofa, watching. "Every day you badger me to eat. And each day I eat something is just another day longer that I'll live. But I don't want to live anymore. I don't want to eat anymore. Okay? It's enough."

They looked at each other a long moment. "Okay," she said.

Dad couldn't get out of bed at all on Tuesday. Grace came over in the morning and put a catheter in. He couldn't urinate anymore. The hospital bed itself had a strong presence in the family room. My dad faded in comparison. I walked to the bed and bent over to kiss his cheek. He smiled weakly. We took turns sitting beside him. When it was my turn, I held his hand.

"I love you, Dad."

"I love you too, honey. Take care of Mom for me."

"I will."

"I'll be waiting for her, you know."

"I know."

On Wednesday, I worked until noon and got to the house by one. He didn't respond anymore. His breathing was noisy, labored. In the family room, Mom stood by his bed, Beth's arm around her back.

"Is this it, then? He won't wake up again?" Tears blurred Mom's eyes as she looked at me.

"Probably not," I answered. I sat down in his La-Z-Boy,

turned it around to face his bed. And rocked. Watched his breathing pattern. After twenty minutes, Mom came back into the room. We switched places, her in the chair. Beth sat on the sofa. Her two daughters stood side by side at the foot of the bed, watching him. Bonnie and her son came and went. Erica floated in and out of the house, made nearly mute by Dad's illness.

Leaf blowers hummed outside. Behind my parents' house I saw a crew with a cherry picker trimming trees around power lines. I remembered that last year around this time, weak from chemo and tired of the crap on TV, he had sat in the living room, watching as workmen cut down a dying tree in the front yard. I thought, at the time, that he seemed pathetic: why didn't he read a book, or listen to books on tape? But he sat there hour after hour, day after day, looking out, watching the crew work their way down the street, trimming tree after tree, pruning the dead branches, demolishing the trunks. It was all he could talk about, all that seemed interesting to him. I listened as his breath came loud and raspy, in an irregular pattern, just irregular enough to keep me listening. He always knew how to hold an audience's attention.

"I think he's gone, you know?" I said. I stared at his profile. "His soul. Sometimes it takes the body a little while to catch up. But it doesn't seem like he's in there anymore."

Beth held a rosary in her hand. "I wondered about that," she said. "Why do you think so?"

"No medical reason. Just a feeling."

As much as I hated seeing him like that, I realized it would ease the transition for us as a family. To see him comatose, to witness the body's ultimate failure would make it easier to let him go. We knew that he didn't want that life for himself. He had made it very clear to all of us.

In the morning, I stopped at the hospital for supplies then drove to my parents' house. I carried the bag inside and set it on the kitchen counter. I said hello to Beth and Mom. They both looked like they hadn't slept in weeks. I picked up the bottle of morphine that Grace had left on top of the microwave oven.

"I'm going to put an IV catheter in him and cap it off," I said. "Not to give him fluids or to feed him. Just so that way we can give him the morphine more directly and not wait until it seems like he's in pain and then give him a shot and wait for it to work."

"I don't know," Beth said. She stood with a hand on Mom's shoulder. They both stared, like they were afraid of me. "Grace said to keep giving him the shots."

"I understand. But subcutaneous absorption is not as reliable as intravenous when the cardiac output is low, which his certainly is. I don't want to see him suffer—nobody wants to. He should not be suffering, regardless of how Grace tells us to do things. This is something I know how to do. If it makes you feel better, I'll put the IV in, and you can page Grace and see what she says. Then we'll give him the morphine when he needs it, but the IV will already be there."

"Are you sure this won't hurt him?" Mom asked. "I don't want you to overdose him."

"I won't," I said grimly. "I'm going to stay here with him the whole time. Nobody has to take responsibility for anything, except me."

I left Beth and Mom in the kitchen. Anesthesia training taught me how to relieve pain. It was the least I could do for him.

After the IV access was in, Beth said, "I talked to Grace. She thinks it's a wonderful idea."

I nodded, counting Dad's respirations. Then slowly gave him the morphine. It should hold him for two to three hours. I counted his respirations again; they were the same after the morphine as before. He'd been taking the medicine for months.

There's lots of discussion in the literature about the "double effect". That means that the drugs we use for pain also sedate people and slow or stop their breathing. Morphine can stop the breathing if you give enough. You have to be careful.

I settled down onto the couch beside the hospital bed. I had brought some magazines, a book to read, various catalogues. Stuff that was piled on top of my desk I hadn't gotten to in weeks. Mail to be gone through, read, thrown out. The regular noise of his breathing sounded almost like a monitor in the operating room. It became a background signal of normalcy that you could ignore until the pattern varied. Periodically, his breathing slowed. I'd look up and wait, watch until I saw the rock of his chest begin again. The body lying there beside me looked nothing like my father, made no sounds like my father, gave me no shit like my father. It was more like a carcass. And though he was never overweight, now all the fat was gone from him. Starvation does that. The small amount of adipose that softens the features, lines the connective tissue, cushions the interface between skin and bones was gone. My father was still a person, but only in the most rudimentary way. His personhood had mostly been eaten up by cancer.

We all stayed with him through the night, rotating every couple of hours. At five, I got up to check on him. The family room was dark, except for a nightlight. Mom sat in a chair she'd pulled up to his bedside, stroking his arm through the bars of the bed. Erica sat on the sofa in her pajamas, head in hand, eyes open and unfocused. Bonnie occupied the La-Z-Boy. I checked Dad's pulse and respirations, drew up a syringe and gave him another dose of morphine. No one looked up or said anything. At six, I drove home to feed the kids breakfast and take them to school. After making the beds and some coffee, I took a shower. As I dressed to go back to my parents', the phone rang.

"It's me," Beth said. "He's gone."

"Just now?"

"Yeah. Grace was here. We were sitting around the table, having cereal, he took a loud deep breath, we looked over, and that was it. He waited till Grace came. Wasn't that just like him?"

I sat on a chair in my bedroom, looking out the window into the yard below. No hint of fall remained. The dead leaves were gone, cleared away by the well-muscled lawn guy. An overcast sky prevented the sun from shining. Relief passed through me, though I wished I'd been there. I didn't know that I needed to be there, I guess, but still, I wished I'd been sitting next to him when it happened. I wished I'd felt it. The loss of life. The transfer of energy. Whatever there was to feel. Even if there's nothing, if that's what it was. But he did it on his own terms. As he had done everything else.

During his first chemotherapy, when Dad cried in my arms, he said he couldn't go through it again. I remember thinking I understood, that I was ready too. I wanted his death to be merciful and quick. But he did go through chemo again. And he lived another year. Over the past few months, when his pain was nearly constant and the things he loved in life were lost to him, I thought I was ready for him to die because it was so hard to watch him suffer. But he stuck it out, much longer than I would have expected, until he stopped eating a few days before. And now I wished he were alive, sitting beside me, telling me some stupid story I'd heard a thousand times.

I remembered the oncologist telling Dad that he wouldn't suffer. He took comfort in that. Of course, it was all crap. Did she just not know? Or is lying easier than telling people the truth? People suffer all the time; they suffer horribly. This should be the great embarrassment for our healthcare system, and instead, untold numbers of American doctors have joined together to pretend it ain't so. But the public knows the truth. Or they sense it. Physicians know the truth. Anyone who has had a loved one die and felt like they were on their own and helpless knows the truth. I am so much luckier than the average person because I understand the medications and know how to relieve pain and am not afraid to do it. And I did it without hastening his death. He died when he chose to.

I'm also lucky because I had a father who showed me something really important—he showed me the value of making plans. As morbid as it seemed, he'd actually done all the preparation he needed to do, long before he needed it. He had created a will and a trust, and he'd given them a lot of thought long ago so that when the time came, he didn't have to explain his wishes to anyone; we didn't have to wonder or discuss it amongst ourselves. His wishes were crystal clear. He made a plan and he stuck with it. I had not given him enough credit. When the end approached, he concentrated on living his life and on his family and his business. He was very clear about what he was willing to put up with. He worked until three weeks before he died because he loved his work and he loved his employees. Then he stopped eating, got into bed, and died five days later. When the time came, he did exactly what he wanted and what he had planned. I felt his incredible determination. All along I'd somehow seen his behavior—the work, the chemo, more work, the unwillingness to let cancer derail him despite his age—as denial, as a failure of logic. But I was wrong: it was my failure to understand that was his strength. The courage he showed was not about chemo or radiation or whether he fought for his life or against his cancer, I hate those similes, but that he got the most out of every single day he could claim as his. *Life is the terminal disease.* How else do you live with that?

# Thirteen

"Are you okay?" my daughter asked the next morning. I'd let Olga in from the yard where she'd celebrated Dad's life by rolling on a dead squirrel. "Ole-gee," he'd called her.

"I can't believe he made it as long as he did."

Bea put her arms around me. Olga stuck her head between us, and her odor brought me back to the present. I said, "I'll take her into town for a shampoo."

An hour and a half later, I parked the car and ran inside the doggy salon to retrieve Olga. Generally speaking, my dog didn't like being coiffed. She started shaking when we were a block away. She whimpered and carried on. A neighbor told me she thought that dog-groomers do weird sexual things to animals, since the dogs seem crazy afterwards. But I figured it was probably something much simpler, like getting soap in their eyes. After I paid, a young girl brought Olga up from the basement on her leash and handed it to me. Sweet Olga, in a near-psychotic frenzy to depart, did a quick lap around my legs. Then the door opened and she made a dash for the great outdoors and freedom. Unfortunately, she caught me off guard, legs still wrapped in leash, and yanked me sideways. Out the door. Down the step. Onto the concrete. With a discreet thud I fell down, landed on a hip and outstretched wrist. The man behind the cash register ran out to assist me.

"Are you hurt?" he asked.

"Oh no," I lied. "I'm fine. Would you mind taking the leash? Then help me up?"

"Sure," he said, looking concerned.

My hip ached, my arm throbbed, my pride was in tatters. But I thought, I'm okay. Then I looked down. My right arm was a completely different shape than my left arm. I frowned.

The young man reached out. "Grab my left arm," I said. He pulled me to my feet.

"Can I drive you home?" he asked.

"Nah, I can drive," I said. "Just put the dog in the back."

I liked Demerol. A lot. It helped the pain. This actually surprised me, even though I'd given gallons of it to patients over the years. I liked the dreamy floating feeling, like giving vague answers on a multiple-choice test. True, false, maybe, sorta, sometimes, whatever. It also got rid of a person's inhibitions. I said whatever came into my mind. Sometimes I lost track of the interiority of my interior monologue. The ER doc, an old friend, had the funniest look on his face, fear almost, a new look for him. It made me laugh. I changed the subject whenever I felt like it. I should have taken it up years ago, like preventive medicine for all of those long and boring discussions on the politics of managed care. A series of doctors came and went. After X-rays, they decided to immobilize my arm and send me to a hand specialist. The orthopedic surgeon told me I might need surgery. And a pin. *F\*\*k that*, I said. I told him surgery was not an option. He had to think of something else, go to Plan B. I was too busy. I needed my right arm. I had things to do. Places to go. Yada, yada. A wake tomorrow, a funeral Monday, a turkey to stuff next Wednesday. Think again.

"Here's what I want," I told him. "I want a nice little waterproof cast, in a somber holiday color, nothing too gaudy, since I've got a funeral tomorrow, so something below the elbow, leaving my fingers free. Okay?"

I heard people whispering. I didn't care. I opened my eyes to see my daughter Bea nodding.

"You're going to see his older partner on Tuesday," she told me. I recognized the technique. A turf, it's called—making me someone else's problem. *Shit*.

In the middle of the night, the pain woke me. I arranged my arm on a pillow, but couldn't get comfortable. The immobilizer covered me from fingers to above the elbow. The arm itched.

I stuck the rounded end of a chopstick down inside to scratch away. I got out of bed to take a couple hydrocodone tablets, then shut myself in the closet, and turned on the light. What clothing did I own with large sleeves, somber enough for a wake, but able to fit over an arm immobilizer? I rummaged around, shoving my throbbing arm inside sleeves from the bottom up so I wouldn't have to take them off the hangers, and eventually found a suit with full sleeves. I opened the drawer with scarves and slips. All silky slippery things together in one place, sliding over themselves. I could take a week's vacation inside my scarf drawer. A pamphlet caught my eye, *How to Tie Scarves*. I sat down on the wooden stool and flipped through the pages. I could use a large scarf as a sling. Something dark. Maybe do a matching eye patch.

Downstairs, I drank a shot of port, then went back to bed. Finally, I fell asleep. I dreamt that I'd driven a very fast car into the country, where I lived on a farm. While planting flowers, I accidentally found human bones. Parts of an old man stuck up through the ground. I told the people who lived on the farm. They sat down on the porch steps and stared at the head and feet of the cadaver. The head was bald, and a yard implement had sliced through part of the scalp. The old man and woman shook their heads and said, "Yup, that's too bad."

~

*Over a year ago, my Dad was told he had cancer, and that it had spread throughout the liver and was in his bones as well. The doctor went on to say that given his age and the fact that his cancer was so advanced, most people wouldn't do anything about it, meaning chemotherapy. My dad was very offended by this. So he found himself a different doctor. Dad was not "most" people.*

*He was a man of many passions. He was passionately in love with my mother, Lydia, his wife of 57 years, he was passionate in his faith in God and the Catholic Church, he was passionate in his devotion to his company and its employees, and he was passionate in his love for his family. He had the utmost respect for the machinists who worked for him; he considered them the foundation of American society. He believed in defending the underdog, though the Cubs and the Bears were notable exceptions, and he always was able to see at least two sides to any issue. He passionately hated Notre Dame. Most particularly he hated their football team. He maintained that no team had a chance against Notre Dame because they had Catholic priests on the sidelines praying for their football team to win. And that offended his sense of fair play. God shouldn't take sides on the football field.*

*As most of you know, Dad had a marvelous sense of humor, which he kept up until the very end, joking with us even from his deathbed. He loved to tell stories, and jokes, and always appreciated hearing a funny story himself. And despite all that, he had an uncanny ability to listen. You knew when you had his full attention, because he would drop his head, purse his lips, and steeple his fingers.*

*Dad knew how to be quiet. He told me once that the secret to his reputation as a highly regarded member of numerous boards and committees was that he hardly ever said a word. Which, he said, was a good thing. Because when he did have something to say, everybody thought he sounded very intelligent. Even when, in his opinion, he was simply pointing out the obvious. That quiet thoughtfulness took him far in life.*

*My earliest memories of my Dad were of sitting on his lap in the early evenings after he came home from work. He read three newspapers every day, the third one being the Chicago Daily News. He taught me to read by running his finger along and reading the words out loud in Mike Royko's column. Then Dad would explain all about "Da Mayor", and how Chicago politics worked, as well*

137

*as how tax assessors were paid off, and how a restaurant got a liquor license in the City of Chicago, and so forth. Then we'd watch Rocky and Bullwinkle and a boxing match or a hockey game. And he'd explain to me the intricacies of boxing or tell me about the history of labor unions. There wasn't much he didn't know about.*

*It has been an amazing privilege for us to watch him manage his illness this past nineteen months. It isn't often in life that we see true courage first hand. We may read about it, or see it dramatized on television, but we rarely glimpse it before our own eyes. And we don't always recognize it right away. Because initially it looks a lot like stubbornness. But over a period of time, Dad's relentless faith in God and in himself and in the people he loved was transformed into something as dogged as any wartime battle. He weighed the risks against the benefits at every step of this journey and made his decisions accordingly. At the age of 81, after having half a lung removed, and a 10 inch steel rod put into his arm to keep the tumor from breaking the bone, and after going through chemo one more time, he went back to work. Carrying his walker, or speeding about the shop in his motorized cart, he continued to look forward, to think about the future of his company, to make certain that his family was cared for. Those were his concerns, up until he died. And that's what we'll remember about him.*

When both my parents were alive, no matter what happened, I had a powerful sense of ballast. You could rock this boat of mine and it would always right itself. But I didn't recognize the force of the stabilizers until they'd gone missing. That sense of solidity, of solidarity, might belong to the category of Rumsfeld's unknown unknowns: you cannot realize what someone provides for you until you make do without. I think strong parents—and a strong family—give you that. Even though I'm the youngest, I speak out as the most observant, the one most inclined to state the obvious. As my father's cancer gradually took him from us, I feared the loss of his stabilizing influence. But it survived him, oddly enough, and made me recognize the strength and power my parents had as a couple. That stayed with us through the twelve additional years that my mother lived. It even endured despite her dementia. But when she died, a familial chasm opened up. I've heard other families remark on the phenomenon. My friend Sam—the second of six—said, "When both our parents died, all hell broke loose." As we gradually fragmented, I wondered if someone could step into that void, fill the symbolic leadership role. Does it work that way? Erica had become ill; Beth lived out of town. Could I do it? Or Bonnie? Or Bonnie and I together? Bonnie was willing to push me to the fore and be my wing-mate. She was willing to do it herself, perhaps, but only with help.

In the year after my mother died, as we mourned and simultaneously dealt with Erica's increasingly complex medical problems, I asked my therapist what to do.

"You do *not* have to be the matriarch," he said to me. "It is your choice. You can say no."

"Really?" It felt like shirking a duty no one had asked me to perform. Similar to pulling weeds. If I do it, they still grow back. And if I don't, it's just a bigger mess.

"Margaret," he leaned forward in his chair. "You do not have to step into these shoes."

"Okay," I said. "I won't." I felt relieved at the time. The shoes were too big, and they'd once been occupied by two people, not one. I had a career and kids of my own. But later on, I found out we were wrong. Someone has to step up. Or pretend to. Practice precedes insight. I didn't have it in me at the time and neither did Bonnie. Or maybe we did, we just didn't want to; we were too tired. Neither my therapist nor I knew what happens when both parents are gone, when there is no captain anymore in a family adrift. The tight flotilla breaks up and what was once a coherent fleet eventually scatters and bobs aimlessly, according to prevailing winds and currents.

# PART FOUR

# Fourteen

Between early March and mid June 2011, I tinkered with ideas, small and large, in my search for a project before returning for my final week at Harvard Business School. I identified problems in the anesthesia department of my hospital, in our surgical areas, and in our workflow; but they seemed either easily fixable with a few changes in policy, or simply not fixable at all given the intransigent personalities involved. I didn't much care. I was part of a huge healthcare machine, a corporate structure that made significant decisions at a level where I didn't function, that didn't seek my input. The decisions that seemed either curious or wrong to me surely made sense to someone somewhere, but I wasn't privy to the rationale or the economics. Designing a business plan for the place I spent my days seemed, paradoxically, like a practical waste of time. There were simply too many hidden and competing agendas, and the problems that concerned me were of a different nature altogether.

What interested me most—*how to manage end-of-life issues in our profit-driven health care environment*—proved too incendiary to take on directly for long periods of time. Though it seemed like a straightforward topic with heft and substance, reading and writing about it felt like tiptoeing over molten lava or staring too long at the sun. I had to take frequent breaks. And so I researched, read and saved articles and books on wildly disparate topics. I dug through stories I'd written in journals and elsewhere about former patients. Instead of seeing only disconnects, I began, steadily, to diagram the linkages.

~

In his essay, "A Good Death", William T. Vollman states, "I will not presume to tell you what death is. Let me content myself with this: There must be better and worse ways to die. It seems both rational and possible to minimize the likelihood of an unpleasant end."[xvii]

So one would hope.

~

I had wanted very much to make my mother's death an easy one. After several years of reflection and research, I am now certain of only one thing: that choice was never mine.

I've seen many bad deaths. I know it is not always possible to avoid bad circumstances, such as a sudden or violent demise. But I wanted to make her comfortable, if that was at all possible. I wanted her to be pain free. I did my best to achieve that end. But even that was not entirely up to me.

~

"You'll take care of me, won't you, Margaret." Two days before her death, in a startling moment of clarity and focus, Mom told me she did not want to die in pain.

She had been in pain for over a month, surprising and gripping but intermittent pain that she couldn't localize or describe. I knew it was staggering by her facial expression. Six weeks earlier, Bonnie had taken her to the doctor, who ordered tests but found nothing. A week later, Vicki called an ambulance. Bonnie and Vicki and I spent most of a day in the ER with Mom as they did scans, drew blood, and tried to determine if something infectious or broken or easily treatable was the cause. All tests came back normal. The ER staff couldn't find anything wrong. Mom, understandably, became more anxious and confused. We took her home with stronger meds. Every day seemed worse than the day before. We'd begun a death vigil, only we didn't know it yet.

Then she couldn't swallow the pills. She stopped eating. She didn't want to drink. Systematically, she began to shut down, to close up shop. I awoke one morning and thought: *I have to put an*

*IV in her in order to give her fluids.* Because I'm an anesthesiologist. That's what I do. I treat people for dehydration and pain and anxiety.

I walked into the locker room at my hospital in late August 2010 where two of my oldest friends and partners, Hayley and Joan, stood changing into scrubs.

"How's your mom, Margaret?" Joan asked.

My eyes filled and I shook my head. "It's not good. The pain medicine isn't holding her. She's getting dehydrated. I'm going to bring home an IV for her."

These strong women reached out to embrace me. I cried harder. Understanding and experience etched both their faces. Joan had lost her mother several years earlier. Hayley's mom had died two years before, and her dad nine months later. "It's time to call hospice," Hayley said gently. "Margaret, let them help you."

I nodded, dumbly. *Of course it was.* Why hadn't I recognized it?

They held onto me for a few moments then let go. I felt a shift occur, a sense of deflation and then a feeling of resolve. I'd spent my adult life advocating for hospice and palliative care. I believe in alleviating pain, in not prolonging suffering in the terminally ill; I believe that people who have expressed their wishes have a right to die on their own terms, in their own time. I believe in doing everything possible to make them comfortable at the end. But even after helping my father, my first inclination was to prolong my mother's life, not ease her way through this passage. I wasn't thinking clearly; I was too close to her. My friends had to remind me.

~

In Vollman's thoughtful essay, written in grief following his own father's passing, he interviews an assortment of "experts" on death: a coroner, a priest, an undertaker, a Baha'i woman, two physicians—all individuals who have experienced many deaths first hand. He attempts to analyze different types of anguish and suffering, to make sense of the journey through them. He differentiates physical from emotional or psychological suffering. This turns out to be an important distinction, one I had not previously considered. It seems so obvious in retrospect.

~

For the first seven of the twelve years that Mom survived Dad, she lived independently in our old family home on the edge of the Elmhurst College campus. She went out with friends, played golf and bridge. She resumed delivering Meals on Wheels and went to Mass every morning. After his death, she took walks and practiced yoga. She lived a surprisingly self-sufficient life. She started to think about moving into a condominium, perhaps a retirement community, but she couldn't muster the resolve to actually do it.

And then she caught the flu. Again. This time she lost her balance. Permanently.

Mom stubbornly continued to play golf. At age eighty-eight, after knocking a ball into the water, she went to retrieve it but she fell, face first, into a creek. She broke her arthritic neck.

The mild dementia she had shown prior to the accident became severe during her two-month hospitalization. We had no way of knowing if it would resolve completely, or what might define her new baseline. And so prior to her discharge from the hospital, we accomplished the change she'd been putting off; we moved her out of her home and into the retirement community where her sister Martha resided, and where she would live out the rest of her life. It was a new environment, not of her choosing. We moved her favorite belongings; we cleaned out her house and eventually sold it. She was not capable of making decisions at that point and, though her decision-making gradually improved over time, it never returned to normal. My sisters and I had the ability to do these things because my dad had transferred the title of their house to us prior to his death. This was, again, part of his estate planning that I came to be grateful for when I took on the role of executor.

~

Several months into my anesthesia residency, I made my way up the stairs to yet another code blue. My intubating skills had improved.

My pager went off again as I emerged from the stairwell through a cold metal doorway, made a right turn, and stopped. Ahead of me stretched a long hall, in the middle of which a shaft of light poured from an office and illuminated a pair of protruding feet. They gave off a red glow. My already pounding heart moved from my chest into my eardrums. I ran forward but cut left through the nursing station and entered the office through the back door.

~

Mom had a newly fused neck from her surgery. She could not turn to look behind her. So her ability to drive—from a physical standpoint—would suffer. At eighty-eight, she already did not drive well. She drove slowly, certainly. But not well. She had not been driving well at eighty-five either. She had recently begun to get lost. And so we took away her car.

~

The female patient lay still on the office floor, completely naked except for her blood, which was everywhere. Bright red blood continued to ooze from her mouth and nose. Beside her, a medicine resident named John sat in a chair with a chart and a sandwich on his lap and stared at her. Blood had splattered his chinos. A year earlier, during internship, John had transferred to me a stroke victim who'd been in the hospital for six months and then died within an hour of transfer, before I got to see him, which made me responsible for dictating a discharge summary for a prolonged hospitalization I knew nothing about.

~

The day in and day out care for a person suffering from dementia is a daunting task. It exhausts, demoralizes, depresses, and overwhelms the caregiver; it is nearly impossible for one person to accomplish alone. Most people require help. My sisters and I shared this burden; the last year of my mother's life we had Vicki, whom we paid out of Mom's savings. We were lucky there was still money with which to pay for home healthcare or it would have come out of our pockets as it does for so many people. Once again, Dad's forward thinking and unrelenting insistence on being prepared for his own and his wife's old age allowed us to provide home care for her.

With the dramatic rise in Alzheimer's dementia,[xviii] with forecasts for huge segments of the population eventually suffering from this horrendous and debilitating disease, and the cost of care skyrocketing accordingly[xix], we have to rethink how we will manage this. Just saving for old age is a luxury few people can afford. Dementia will soon become a national health disaster. Up until now, patients typically have been kept at home, with care being loosely strung together by families who hire caregivers or utilize adult daycare when they can't provide coverage. Institutions have been an expensive alternative of last resort. The possibility of living with dementia looms big in my mind: I hope never to be a burden to my children. I don't think they owe me that. But at the same time, what are my options? I had a patient who attempted suicide after being given a diagnosis of Alzheimer's. I had a therapist who bought a gun.

~

"Where's the crash cart?" I asked John. No way was I giving mouth to mouth through a geyser of blood.

"It's not here yet," he answered. "I called for it."

"Do you know this patient?" A nurse pushed a cart with emergency equipment into the room. I grabbed a mask and ambu bag off the side, hooked it to the oxygen tank and tried to put it on the patient's face. I felt completely alone in my sense of urgency.

"Yes, I do. She had esophageal cancer, and irradiation. I think her cancer eroded into her aorta."

"Are there any gloves?" I asked the nurse.

"I don't see any," she answered, glancing around.

~

My mother declined rapidly and significantly during her last year. She lost her spark, her energy, and her appetite. She stopped recognizing people she'd known all her life. She remembered Bonnie and me, as she saw us most frequently, but she lost my other sisters and all her grandchildren. She went from riding the exercise bike to barely rising from a chair. If someone asked me in November 2009, as a physician, do you expect this person— your mother—to be alive in a year, I would have said *No*. That is a powerful diagnostic tool, as it turns out. I did not expect her to survive that long. And I was right; she did not.

I don't exactly know what caused my mother to die, except that she was really old. But *old age* isn't something to write on a death certificate. Not officially, anyway. According to Sherwin Nuland's excellent book on the subject, *How We Die*, in real life we see it happen. All the body's systems seem to slow down and the body just gradually quits; we find something else to write for documentation purposes. My mother stopped eating. She stopped getting out of bed. She became weak. Mom might have had some combination of pathological processes, but I don't know what they were. Her abdomen grew larger, or else she shrank in height; there wasn't any sign of ascites or a mass. She may have had inadequate blood flow to her intestines from aging arteries. It might have been something entirely different. She had pain, which seemed to originate from the back and come around to the front, but she could never describe it or localize it; it just gripped her and then let her go. I've read this is common in dementia[xx]. But because she was in pain, we gave her pain medicine.

In the truly old, it seems as though the life force comes to an end; there's a turning inward of energy and spirit. The opposite of unfurling. I don't know how else to describe it. But what's surprising and disheartening about that process was that it was so painful for her. You would think that dying of old age should be something from which you simply slip away, like my hundred-year-old patient Esther. But my mother was not that lucky.

~

"Is she DNR?" I knelt down on the floor near the patient's head. Blood soaked through my pants. I placed a mask on her face but it kept slipping off. She didn't have any teeth, and it's difficult to mask ventilate someone without teeth. The blood made it nearly impossible. "*Is she DNR?*" I repeated. Why would John be sitting there watching a person bleed to death?

"I'm checking the chart."

"Shouldn't we be doing CPR? Just in case?"

"There's no point, really, she doesn't have any blood left to push around with chest compressions." He flipped through pages while I blew bubbles into the blood around her face with the ambu bag. "Here it is. Yes, she is DNR. Do Not Resuscitate. *Excellent.*"

~

In the period between 1998 and 2010—the twelve years that spanned my parents' deaths—admissions to hospice grew dramatically, as did the number of organizations providing hospice care. Expenditures for the Medicare benefit for *hospice* expanded from $2.2 billion in 1998 to $12.1 billion in 2009. The number of conditions for which hospice could be utilized was expanded, and the length of stay trended upward until it peaked in 2006. It has dropped slightly since then. It is difficult to determine how much money has been saved by a corresponding decline in hospitalization costs for these patients, but the estimate is that hospice care runs approximately one third of in-hospital costs.

I'm the type of person who usually does a lot of comparison shopping. It may take me months to buy a coffee maker, a year to purchase a car. But I'm embarrassed to admit that it never occurred to me to shop for hospice agencies. We signed up for one when my dad needed it, and we got very lucky. Grace took incredible care of my father and of us, and the whole process felt effortless. But in the twelve years between my parents' deaths, hospice became big business.

~

I leaned back on my heels, nearly as covered in blood as the dead lady. I looked at John in amazement. "Why'd you call a code?" I asked. "If you knew or thought she was *Do Not Resuscitate*, why did you call it?"

"I wanted to see how fast you'd get here," he said, and then he laughed.

~

We utilized two separate hospice organizations for my parents, and the differences between them were dramatic. The hospice we utilized in 1998 was a small organization that operated through a community hospital, and we dealt with one nurse over a period of about two and a half weeks. In my mother's case, we contracted the hospice through the retirement community where she resided. Hospice was involved for just under a month before she died. We met at least seven nurses during that time; the only one who I met more than once came the last three days of Mom's life. And the final nurse—the death nurse, if you will—was great. But I have nothing good to say about the rest of the organization. I wrote letters after her death, to no avail. So I recommend doing your homework before deciding on a hospice provider; don't take the first one offered out of convenience or implied contractual obligation. This is an important decision; make it carefully.

~

Vicki expressed her deep opposition to hospice and to morphine; in her mind, morphine meant certain death. I understood that morphine frightened her. But death was already certain, and my mother's pain frightened me more. I tried to explain to Vicki that Mom needed morphine because she approached death, not the other way around. But the fear stayed with Vicki. To me, morphine is just a drug; I feel comfortable with drugs. Because of my job, I understand them. I could not do anything about my mother's age; I could not reverse the changes that time had wrought. But with the help of hospice and medication we could make her final days bearable.

Only in retrospect have I come to understand what *bearable* means. Like *suffering*, the word itself contains implied elasticity.

~

I knelt on the floor and stared at the dead woman whose sudden exsanguination had, with minimal preamble, closed the book on whatever manner of times she'd known—good, bad, tedious, tragic, with the likely long stretches of fretting that define a life for the average woman. This was an *awful* death, I thought, and not just because she was naked on the cold floor covered in blood in an equally hard-hearted environment. But the last person she saw was this asshole, *John*. She made the mistake of getting out of her bed to ask for help and found him instead.

~

When we were near the end, when Mom stopped eating and drinking, when she could no longer get out of bed, we called Beth to come from Florida. Erica was visiting daily, and her kids came as often as they could. I called my daughter Ruthann in Georgia. Bea lived with me at the time, and made regular visits to see Mom.

When Beth arrived, she told me that she felt comfortable with my giving Mom morphine to ease her passage, since she was in pain and clearly at the end of her life. She had been with me when I had done the same for Dad. In the interim, she had done some research on the matter and had come to the conclusion that giving morphine to a terminally ill person to relieve their suffering is humane. The palliative care literature refers to the administration of opioids and benzodiazepines, when given with the intent of relieving suffering and not hastening death, as the *double effect*, as they may cause sedation which is both ethically and legally sanctioned[xxi]. The priest from Mom's church had already given her last rites.

~

Vollman quotes a Buddhist chaplain who says that most people die the minute someone leaves the room. Vollman states, "I think that when my time comes I will seek to die alone."

~

The hospice intake worker had told us we could expect a visit from their chaplain, who showed up on the afternoon of September 21st, 2010.

He introduced himself, shook hands, then asked if we had any particular requests.

Beth glanced around at the rest of us—Vicki, Erica, Bonnie and me. "I think it would be nice if you could say the Lord's Prayer." I nodded.

"I don't do the Lord's Prayer," he said. "But I sing."

Vicki stood at the end of the bed, anxiously wringing her hands and ready to cry. I was kind of glad Mom was comatose at that moment. *He didn't do the Lord's Prayer?* I looked at Beth who was biting her lower lip and trying not to laugh. Erica gazed into her own lap with a horrified frown. Bonnie couldn't look up; her face was contorted as she tried to control her expression. I almost wished Dad were there. He would have thrown the guy out. The chaplain, sporting a ridiculous hairpiece, burst into song, much like a musical theater buff who'd randomly crashed our death party. *What kind of chaplain refuses to say the Lord's Prayer?* There was nothing comforting about hearing him sing hymn after hymn although he seemed to be enjoying himself.

*"Please, just stop,"* Beth said to him after the sixth song sung off-key. *"Really! Please. That's enough...singing. Thank you."* I guess, in retrospect, he lightened the mood, though I don't think that was his intention.

~

"Well, it's dinnertime," John said, tossing his blood-splattered sandwich into a garbage can. "Think I'll go get some chow. You're welcome to practice tubing her, if you want. Since she's dead and you're a mess." He spun his desk chair around and wrote something in the chart. I took deep breaths of the rusty air and shut the patient's eyes with my thumbs. A few people showed up, belatedly, to the aborted code blue but were waved away. I climbed to my feet and struggled to keep my balance on the slippery floor. The nurse threw down a towel so that I could wipe my shoes.

~

Mom died the day after the chaplain came to sing at us, after we'd said our own prayers. I phoned Gibbons Funeral Home to make the arrangements; within twenty minutes we'd covered all necessary details. Then I rushed out of Mom's condo and sped downtown to see my therapist who had kept my time open in case I needed it. It all seems odd to me now, in retrospect, how much I needed it. I felt completely bereft but said little during my hour. He hugged me when I got up to leave.

# Fifteen

I returned to Cambridge for my final session of *Managing Healthcare Delivery* in June 2011. The third module focused on creating and fostering an innovative, learning organization. Our business plans were due before we arrived. I drew up an outline for a book, but didn't turn it in. I had only begun to do the research and realized how much I had yet to learn.

The Harvard Business School approach to fixing modern healthcare involves deconstructing what works in various organizations, environments and markets and using that knowledge to try to reconstruct success in different scenarios. They employ some of the smartest people in the country who've already had incredible success in business and (even) government and now want to share their knowledge. We learned from them about the elements of that success, what drives and sustains it, and what disrupts it. What are the potential problems and reasons for failure? Where do breakdowns in communication occur and how does that get translated in our workplace? Fluidity is important. Culture can be a big problem in healthcare as in other industries; changing it sometimes requires new leadership, sometimes it requires complete redesign. Taking a systems approach—while critical—must be balanced against maintaining the direct responsibility of individuals in a high-reliability organization. In medicine, we learn a lot about safety from the airline industry and NASA. We learn from their analysis of errors, from their culture, from the ways they succeed. We strive to create an environment of zero mistakes. We fail miserably and it makes us try harder. Healthcare requires the identification of strong leaders, leaders who support and foster growth and new ideas. The days of iron-fisted rulers, people like Dr. Cruzario from my internship days, who issue dictums but abandon individual patients, are over. A good leader is one who fosters new ideas, encourages people to speak up, and creates an environment that allows for growth. Physicians can make good leaders, but they rarely do; being a good physician traditionally has had nothing to do with leadership. Doctors aren't paid to lead, nor do they typically have the opportunities to develop those skills. But successful medical systems actually need everyone to be successful, from bottom to top. Harvard teaches an approach that looks at large organizations that can reach large numbers of customers and do it in a sustainable fashion. It is not a public health program; it is a business school model. It does not concern itself with every uninsured American; it looks at well-run systems and how to replicate them in smaller markets. It is not everything to all people. It doesn't try to be.

Fundamentally, the case study method consists of little more than applied storytelling. The professors delivered their messages in tidy bundles for discussion purposes. Later they imparted the less tidy truths about the all-too-human leadership, the less-than-ideal marketplace, the foibles that interfered with the scripted and concise successes. Stories only told part of the story.

It gradually occurred to me that business schools depend on the revenue generated by their Executive Education programs. It must be a difficult course to navigate, when their research seems to suggest that healthcare in countries with single-payer systems works better than what we have here in the U.S. with our free market, insurance based system. And how do you draw profit-driven enrollees from that system to your course, when the tuition is substantial? You may have some really astute answers to the difficult questions that plague healthcare providers and administrators, but you can't present them as such. Because not everyone wants to hear them. Rather, you have to pose them instead as just the right questions, in just the right ways, so that the students are left to draw their own conclusions. Then you hope they will be on board. You have to accept there will be some who don't buy what you're selling, others who will drink your Kool-Aid, and still others who have missed the point entirely. You will change the lives of a few.

I'd read an article by Louis Menand in the January 24, 2011 issue of *The New Yorker* called "Books as Bombs: Why the women's movement needed the *Feminine Mystique*". To me the power of the article was not just about feminism, it was the idea that social change occurs when the time is right. The more I learned about healthcare, the less I believed that the necessary bedrock changes would occur as a result of legislative efforts. Whatever came out of Congress would be hopelessly watered down, subjected to debilitating compromise and rendered marginally effective by endless bureaucracy. The country has become too political, too polarized. And those who lack healthcare don't have powerful lobbying groups to represent their interests. So how do we chip away at massive, yet simultaneously inadequate, healthcare expenditures? How do we improve just one small part of healthcare? Rhetoric, in and of itself, is the strong arm tactic of the enemy.

I relaxed during my final week at Harvard and took in as much as I could. I socialized more, went out for drinks and dinner with other students. It was springtime in Boston and I walked along the Charles each day. My grief had begun to abate.

At the end of our week, many students presented their business plans. Some of these presentations were ways to expand private practices, or the presenters' own personal businesses. Others were plans to improve services lines in their organizations. Some groups got together to demonstrate how their shared learning could be useful for their organizations in concrete ways to expand product lines, improve facilities, and so on. For some it was revenue generating, for others it was reducing expenses and becoming more profitable.

But my interest centered round the experiences of my past, particularly the thirteen years I'd spent caring for two elderly parents. My thoughts kept coming back to care at the end of life. How do we change the end game? How do we make it better for the elderly, for those of us who will some day become elderly, and how do we save our country some money in the process so that when it is our turn, there will be money left in the system to provide us with the care we want? It seemed to me that if we could just tinker with this one aspect of healthcare, a number of other issues would fall into place.

When I arrived home from Boston in June 2011, I had certainly learned a lot about healthcare management.

I no longer believed that legislation alone could provide the answers. I no longer believed that the healthcare industry would provide the answers. Whenever there is profit to be made in healthcare, be it by a pharmaceutical company, an insurance company, a hospital, a physician group, or any combination of the myriad of affiliated industries, any single patient's or individual's best interest—a complex concept that will vary over the course of that person's lifetime—must be determined by that *individual* or his guardian, perhaps only guided by individual physicians along the way. As long as someone stands to profit from the propagation of health services, which may or may not improve your life most particularly at the end of your life, you cannot trust that you will receive sound advice. Even Mother Teresa had an agenda.

So what are the options?

Well, it's complicated.

If we were to collect all the data, study it, then take a good hard look at how people say they want to die and how the laws currently dictate that they will die unless they state otherwise, society as a whole would turn the tide of our current healthcare trend and demand better treatment for itself, which is to say, fewer procedures, less "treatment", and more "care". Most of us would pay closer attention to getting the most out of every remaining day instead of spending our time trying desperately to stay alive. This is the current thrust behind the growing palliative care movement in the United States. An excellent and thorough resource guide for physicians caring for terminally ill patients is the compendium of case studies published by the Journal of the American Medical Association, *Care at the Close of Life: Evidence and Experience.*[xxii]

Patients, unfortunately, have miserable deaths all the time. Though I felt strongly that I had kept Mom as comfortable and as pain-free as was humanly possibly, I also know that what when I said, *My mother died in hospice*, it wasn't strictly true. My mother died in a stylized, personalized version of hospice, brought to her by my very compulsive, pharmacologically knowledgeable self. So the question remains: Is there any way to die that isn't painful without a committed and loving health care professional at your bedside?

I think there is, but it requires thought, planning, and probably an element of luck.

Dr. Angelo Volandes from Massachusetts General Hospital has created a series of short videos that serve as adjuncts to decision making for those pondering end of life choices[xxiii]; the videos provide nonverbal illustrations of dementia, CPR, and other end-stage clinical situations that can be difficult to adequately describe *verbally*. These three minute videos have been adopted by many healthcare systems as educational tools; they are not available for individual use, but the website gives a reasonable sample of their calm and clear explanations. The goal of Volandes' *Advance Care Planning Decisions* video tool is not to save money, though that would be a natural outcome of reducing excessive and unwanted end-of-life care, but rather it is to educate people and help them plan appropriately while they are still able.

The current medical system worked for my parents, more or less. It worked for my dad because he had the foresight to choose what he wanted, to stay at home, to use hospice, and to decide when he was going to stop eating. He did so and died. He was in control. Yes, he had a surgical procedure during the final three months of his life—the rodding of his humerus to stabilize the bone for pain and to prevent fracture. He was hospitalized less than twenty-four hours; his physician performed the procedure prophylactically. Could he have done without? Possibly. He had radiation as well for the control of pain. All of that cost money that, in retrospect, might have been wasted. Dad and his doctor made educated guesses, erring on the side of "safety" and more care—the traditional mindset of a fee-for-service system. My mother had one hospitalization ten months before her demise, and one emergency room visit six weeks prior to death. Dementia made her treatment far more daunting, her care more confusing. We spent a lot of money, as did Medicare Part D, on the dementia medication *Aricept* that did her no good whatsoever. But the pharmaceutical industry certainly profited.

In a *Lancet* article[xxiv] from 2011, Harvard researchers found that among 1.8 million Medicare beneficiaries who died in 2008: nearly one in three had surgery in the last year of life; nearly one out of five had surgery in the last month of life; nearly one out of ten had surgery in the last week of life. Those are astounding numbers. Of course many of those procedures were performed to relieve suffering or to prolong life. But did they? The researchers said they know from experience—as all of us do in eldercare—that doctors often operate to fix something that will not save a dying patient, and in doing so *avoid* the difficult conversations with patients and caregivers about their prognosis and what they want.

As patients, our legal rights have been fairly limited. If you do not want to be given fluids or food because you feel, as my dad felt, that it was only feeding his cancer, then do not go to the hospital and do not let someone take you there. Even if you have a living will, even if you are *Do Not Resuscitate*, you will be given those things. Make your wishes known earlier rather than later; fill out all the paperwork your state requires. Have the hard discussions with your loved ones today. Don't wait. Later on they may prevail upon your physicians to withdraw support, but support will be instituted first unless you specifically refuse, which is no easy task. Withdrawing support is much different than never starting it in the first place. And asking someone, even or especially a close relative, to refuse all treatment on your behalf is asking a lot. Many people choose to stay home. End of life care is a slippery slope; these issues are worth thinking about and talking about ahead of time. See the Compassion and Choices website for an excellent values worksheet that will get you thinking about what you really want and that can help guide you through a discussion with your loved ones.

# Sixteen

One Wednesday in July 2011, I sat in my therapist's office and told him I would not be coming back. I needed to pursue the life I'd been contemplating; I needed to finish my business plan. I suspected that several issues might grow clearer outside the safety of the room with the beautiful view of our great city.

"I think I'm done," I told him. "This head is shrunk."

He seemed concerned by my decision and asked me why.

"Well, I've come to think of this as a friendship, but I know I'm not your friend. So it feels unbalanced this way. I bring you existential problems or think of stories to create a conversation, just to hear what you have to say. That isn't right. That's paying for something that should be free and a normal part of my life." Therapy had become either a credit or a debit, but not something I could locate on either side of the T-bar.

I acknowledged the important and difficult work we had done together, and thanked him for helping me through some very hard times. He had been an excellent guide through the harrowing maze of my psyche; I emerged with a better and richer understanding of every trauma I'd survived. But more importantly, he had taught me to embrace my cognitive dissonance, not to deny it or pathologize it. Rather, I accepted it as defining my way of inhabiting the world, like being a gassy baby or having a twitchy eye. Like my father, I was good at problem solving and managing complexity. Cognitive dissonance might even be considered my gift. It is a constant reminder that I will never wear lemon juice, even on days when it would feel really good; I know I don't know things and I will spend my life trying to learn them. Just as the astrologer had mentioned. Still, I would miss my therapist. He believed in me, and for a long time I had counted on him for that.

Later that summer, my sisters and I rented a beach house in Southwestern Michigan for a few weeks. Beth and her husband Andrew, Bonnie, our kids, their partners, their kids, and some friends all came and stayed for part or all of the time. Erica, due to ongoing health issues, couldn't join us. My dog Olga shared the basement bedroom with me for the final week of the rental; she no longer climbed stairs. We had a separate kitchen where I cooked her three daily meals of hamburger with buns. It was the first time our family had been together since Mom's passing.

I walked the beach in the mornings. This corner of Michigan summons cyclists from the entire Midwest so I rode my bicycle every day, thirty or forty miles along country roads, stopping to take pictures of cows and barns and old farm equipment. Sometimes you don't realize how much you need a vacation until you pedal along a quiet back road alone with your thoughts and your headphones screaming alternative rock.

Remembering what the astrologer had told me, I looked at real estate. I realized I liked being out of Chicago, away from the noise of the city. Some money that my parents left allowed me to make a down payment on an old cottage in the woods in Harbor Country, about eighty-five miles from Chicago. The investment would force me to save, as well as provide my daughters and me with a year-round retreat; we could hike and bike, garden, go to the beach, read, and relax.

I feel my parents' spirits in Michigan and know they would have been happy to sit on my screened porch and read the newspaper or just gaze at the hummingbirds in the garden. The cottage has given me something I didn't know I needed, which is a family home. I have finally regained my ballast; I find the quiet that I miss by living in the loud and frenetic city. I'm able to harness the power of intention and concentration that long periods of hard work in the medical environment consistently drain from me. I get my energy back when I go to the woods, walk the beach, and bike the country roads. After all, I am an introvert with an eye on the big picture, a storyteller interested in the senescent cells of progeroid mice, an Aries who reads the horoscope of a Taurus. During my foray at business school, I learned that stories can be used both to illustrate and to obfuscate. I also learned that suffering makes us who we are, which explains why there are so many different types of suffering.

Buying the cottage has given my family a place to gather, should one of my sisters or I decide to become a matriarch after all. We argue over who will get that thankless job. I suppose we are all matriarchs of a sort already: my daughters believe that I know how to fix things, how to choose a ripe melon, and how to make a frittata from whatever might be left in the fridge. I find myself learning from them too: Bea teaches me about car maintenance and nutritious cooking; Ruthann instructs me in yoga and how to date. Ironically, they insist that we "juice" on our weekends together. I keep the lemons well away from them.

During the 2012 winter, our beloved Olga grew frail and weak. She came from the Humane Society fifteen years earlier after she'd been taken and then returned by another family. A noble mix of Greyhound and German Shepherd, Olga had the personality of the hound—sweet and gentle, a loving leaner.

"Where did you get her?" strangers in the park would often ask.

"From the Humane Society..."

"Oh, so you *rescued* her," came the typical retort.

Well, sure, I suppose I did. But I hate the insinuation of the term; just because I got a dog for free doesn't mean I'm a generous person. In fact it had more to do with a belief in Darwinian theory and the strength of a broad genetic pool than any intrinsic goodness on my part. I wanted a mutt because I thought she'd be healthier. As it turned out, she rescued me.

But by early winter of 2012, she was no longer healthy, no longer strong. The bad days outnumbered the good ones. She no longer rose to greet me when I came home from work. She only ate a little even when she was hand fed; her legs routinely gave way on our slow walks. She was suffering; Bea, Ruthann and I discussed it with Jeremy, our dog walker, who had taken care of her for the past six years.

When the movie *Marley and Me* was released a few years ago, Bea told me not to see it. She said, "Mom, you can't handle a movie like this. DO NOT see this movie. Seriously, you'll sob. I started crying about ten minutes into it, and cried the whole way through, because I knew how it was going to end."

I took her advice. I didn't see the movie.

When Olga and I went to see her vet, Marco, for a check-up one day, I asked him if he'd seen it.

"Yes, I saw that movie. The whole movie I said to myself, *so train the dog already!* Margaret, you would watch eet and 'chew would say to yourself, *'wat ees the matter with these people that they don't train their dog?* If it was us, we would train the dog. 'Ees ridiculous! Of course, I sobbed at the end."

With two people I trusted giving me advice, I avoided that movie like heartworms.

And then in the winter of 2009, I tore my rotator cuff and had it repaired a couple of months later. Ruthann came home for a few days to help me out, and while I was recuperating from the surgery we watched a lot of movies. I can only blame the *Oxycontin* for the lapse in judgment that led me to believe that we should watch *Marley and Me*.

Of course, it is a ridiculous movie. It is all about how people did not bother to train their dog. As my marvelous companion Olga lay on the floor beside me, snoozing away, I shook my head and commented—in a drug-induced state—on the kind of idiots that would allow an untrained dog to have complete access to their house. Hadn't they heard of crates? There were lots of methods to train dogs. Why, Olga had won most improved in her puppy class the first time, and then again when we went back for a remedial round.

My dog never sat on the furniture, I smugly thought to myself. My dog doesn't sniff crotches. My dog doesn't tear up upholstery...

On the other hand, if I remembered correctly, as I watched the movie, it occurred to me that pretty much every crime that *Marley* committed had been equaled or surpassed by Olga. Busting through a screen to chase a squirrel? Hmm, yup. Tearing apart her puppy bed in less than thirty minutes? That too. We had some dramas and miracles of our own with Olga, such as the time she took out my knee and I had to have an ACL reconstruction. Or when I broke my wrist after Dad died. Or the time she took off after a bird and was hit by a Chicago city bus but somehow survived. A Chicago Fire Department chief and I had to crawl on our stomachs under the bus on a frigid March morning, pass a flattened cardboard box beneath the dog, and drag her out. A total stranger loaned me a jacket to wear; I'd run outside in a panic. The girls and I drove Olga to the emergency room on Clybourn Avenue where the vet declared her shocky but stable. She had no broken bones. Afterwards we coaxed her into the elevator for her daily walks; it took some time to overcome a not-irrational fear of bus noises.

And I stopped making fun of *Marley and Me*.

Marco came to the house to give Olga her final shot on a cold evening in February. She had advanced arthritis. And so she passed with her favorite people holding onto her, at her favorite spot on the carpet, just outside my bedroom door.

We had been through everything together, Olga and I. When I lived alone, she slept beside me. When Bea moved home, she slept in the hallway between us. All along, I believed somehow that she felt my pain. And finally, in the last few months, I felt hers. That was how I knew it was time to let her go somewhere else—someplace where her joints wouldn't hurt, where there was lots of fresh pee to sniff, and maybe my mom to lean against and beg cookies from. I hope that's where she is now. I was so grateful I could help her that way. It was *humane*. I stopped her suffering. Maybe she's making friends with a cheesy Lab movie star named Marley.

Of course, people aren't dogs. We treat dogs better than we treat people.

The year before my father died, I had to put down an English Bulldog named Fergie. I sat with her while the vet gave her the final injection and cried my eyes out. She lived only four and a half years. Bulldogs have a ridiculous number of medical problems, which is one of the reasons I chose a mutt when I went looking for Olga. The week after I had Fergie euthanized, the vet sent me a handwritten note: a lovely, heartfelt acknowledgment of how difficult it is to make a decision like I had on behalf of my suffering pet. But he felt I'd done the right thing. I cried all over again, but I never doubted that my decision was correct.

A few weeks after losing my father, I ran into his oncologist at a hospital event. She never said a word to me. She didn't say, "I'm sorry for your loss," or "How is your dad?" She pretended she didn't know him or me or that she'd ever uttered those hideous words to him, "You won't suffer."

But we can keep people from suffering. Or we can tell them the truth about how much suffering there will be and let them make up their own minds at each step along the way. We don't have to profit from their pain. That would be the humane thing to do. And as patients, we can take a stance that we aren't willing to suffer, that we will hold healthcare professionals accountable who promote suffering in the name of longer lives, or "your only option". There is always another option, and that might be to do nothing but relieve the pain and say good-bye. The Study to Understand Prognoses and Preferences for Outcomes and Risks of Treatments (SUPPORT) found that fifty percent of patients who were conscious at the end had moderate to severe pain at least half the time in the last three days of the their lives. DNR orders were written two days before death forty-six percent of the time. Only forty-seven percent of patients' physicians knew what their preferences were with respect to DNR[xxv]. That is poor communication, poor planning, and way too much lemon juice on a very large scale.

Suffering is one complex, difficult question that you must break down into smaller, easier questions in order to tackle properly. You must do this knowingly, without the application of lemon juice. It helps to use stories to illustrate suffering, because otherwise we pretend it will not happen to us. Stories promote empathy. Abstraction does not. People's narratives and patients' experiences taught me this: when you abstract suffering, you lose touch with the individual and you stop caring. And the cost of that will be unaffordable.

I sat at dinner one evening with an old friend and said, "I started out thinking this book was about writing advance directives. That a large part of the healthcare crisis could be averted if people just gave a little thought to what they want at the ends of their lives, and make their wishes known to their loved ones. Fill out a couple of forms. But the more I get into it, the more I realize it isn't that simple. And I keep going further afield."

We were at a restaurant in a suburb north of Chicago. Having tacos and a beer. She said, "Well you know I'm an *Exit Guide*."

Uh no, I didn't know that.

Soon I learned about the old Hemlock Society, its rebirth in the 1990's as two separate entities: Compassion and Choices, a national organization that provides *invaluable* education, information, and help with regard to end-of-life care, and the Final Exit Network, which is an organization that provides help with assisted suicide for the terminally ill. I joined the Chicago End of Life Coalition. I learned about the states that have death with dignity legislation in place, passed by referendum in Washington and Oregon, and Vermont, where the legislature voted in 2013 to allow "dying, mentally competent people determine when they have endured enough suffering and empowers them to end their lives with dignity. Specifically, it will provide criminal, civil and professional protections for physicians who prescribe medication to mentally competent, terminally ill patients that they can ingest to achieve a peaceful death"xxvi. The California legislature followed suit in 2015, with an assisted-suicide law going into effect January 1st, 2016. To a similar end, the Montana Supreme Court ruled in 2009 in a case brought by Compassion & Choices, *Baxter v. Montana*, that the state's public policy supports mentally competent, terminally ill patients being able to choose aid in dying.

Naturally, controversy swirls around organizations like Final Exit Network here and Dignitas in Switzerland. Organized medicine looks askance at involving physicians in end of life transitions. *Frontline* did a piece that brought some particular issues into question, focusing on the deaths of individuals who were shown not to have terminal illnesses. The show was meant to be an indictment of the Final Exit Network, but when I discussed it the next day with people at the hospital, there was a huge amount of support for the work it does, perhaps because such a tremendous need exists. In medicine, we see how much suffering occurs at the end of life. Personally, I am glad to know that these resources exist, should I need one some day. It's hard to know what the future holds. And I am glad to know an Exit Guide; I am happy that someone will help me if I am terminally ill and suffering. Maybe by that time we will have more than a handful of states with physician-assisted suicide.

My sojourn at Harvard Business School happened to coincide with a period of profound personal grief. I came to understand that grief sharpens acuity. For this reason, my world coalesced in a strange and particular way; the grief galvanized my thoughts and emotions and spurred me to take a fresh, hard look at what had become commonplace medical practice. The profit motive remains a powerful and insidious reason to extend life at all costs, without concern for quality for either patients or their families. I couldn't help but come to an important conclusion: *capitalism* had ruined healthcare. But did capitalism ever belong in healthcare in the first place? It certainly does not belong in death and dying. If you accept that, then you take a somewhat different look at healthcare. You slowly back up from the end of life, incrementally evaluating American delivery systems in all their permutations. You back up from extreme illness toward not-so-extreme illness, toward moderate illness and chronic disease to wellness and simple aging. And you try to imagine where capitalism should be inserted, into which phase of your life's medical care the profit motive should be suddenly placed. I'm not sure I see the pivot point, the point where it suddenly makes sense.

Generations of physicians have been educated in this system and it will take a strong public outcry to demand change. Only recently has the palliative care movement begun to take hold in various parts of our country; it appears to be surging at a rapid rate. It is up to patients to take control over their health and wellbeing, and especially their deaths, to ask questions, and to make their own plans.

Taking control gives you choices that come only with knowledge. The array of unknown unknowns narrows as you learn about your health, as you broaden your base of medical knowledge. Denial, as they say, isn't just a river in Egypt. It is the deadliest form and application of lemon juice that exists.

I have read Vollman's essay many times over. It contains much wisdom. Though my mother's death was painful, I do not believe that she *suffered*. Mom wasn't afraid. And she wasn't unhappy. Her loved ones surrounded her. Bonnie and I, Beth and Erica, her grandchildren, Vicki in particular, all tended to her during her final weeks. I did my best to ease her physical pain. I suspect, had we ever left the room, she might have slipped away more quickly, more gently into the night. But we never gave her the chance because we never left her alone.

As for my own personal wishes, well, if I drop dead tomorrow, and a defibrillator happens to be hanging nearby, go ahead and put the paddles on. Give me a shock or two, if I need it.

Unexpected death can be successfully reversed often enough to make it worth a try. But if I wave you away, if I'm chronically ill and lingering, let me go. Those are my wishes. If I've developed dementia, don't put a feeding tube in me. Don't put me on a ventilator; don't take me to the operating room. Don't transplant any organs into me; save them for the young people who need them. Take me home, give me some morphine, let me have some time on my screened porch to say my good-byes; just make me comfortable and let me go. I've had a good life; I've puzzled my way through my dissonance and not a drop of lemon juice is in sight anymore. In case there's some confusion about the matter, please see my legal documents where everything is explained in detail. My children know where to find them.

My business plan eventually morphed into a book, *this book*, which I will now bring to its conclusion. Hopefully, it emphasized the value of making your own plans; start small but start somewhere. If we all do it, the effect will be huge.

# Afterword

I want to thank my wonderful daughters for their love and support throughout the arduous process of writing this book. As always, they keep me sane and balanced. They encourage me; they take me out for walks when I've been too long indoors. They make sure I eat vegetables on occasion.

Much gratitude goes to my sisters and other family members for sharing memories and insights. Nick, the hours you've spent on our ancestry are deeply appreciated.

I am particularly beholden to my many friends, but particularly Janet Desaulniers, Karen Schneider, Jane Dale, Claudia Johnson, and Patrick Toomay for believing in the importance of the topic as well as my ability to deliver the goods. I wasn't always so sure. You guys propped me up. So many friends and acquaintances wanted to talk about this subject while I was writing that I felt encouraged by their interest.

I am deeply grateful to my fellow anesthesiologists at what was formerly known as PRAA for your ongoing support and amazing willingness to share stories and experiences. Our many discussions about work and life and accumulated years of practice fueled much of what enabled me to write this story. Your skills, your outrage, and your empathy continue to make me believe in the best aspects of American medical care and in the integrity of the American physician. I also want to thank the many nurses, physician assistants, technicians, surgeons, gastroenterologists, and various medical and ancillary personnel who shared their stories with me. And Patrick Fanning, of course, for reading and for allowing it to happen.

Thank you sweet Olga.

And finally, most importantly, thank you Lydia and Carl. *For everything.*

# Endnotes

[i] Samuel Shem, *The House of God*, Berkley Publishing, 1978.

[ii] Meyers Briggs Type Indicator is a personality inventory derived from the psychological types described by Jung which predicts preferences in perception and judgment. Sixteen distinctive personality types are described.

[iii] Dan P. McAdams, *The Redemptive Self: Stories Americans Live By*. New York, NY: Oxford University Press, 2006.

[iv] Cognitive dissonance refers to psychological discomfort resulting from conflicting ideas, beliefs, and values held simultaneously.

[v] Cooper, et al., "Cardiopulmonary Resuscitation: History, Current Practice, and Future Direction," *Circulation*. 2006; 114: 2839-2849.

[vi] Please see original article for complete details: Dunning, et al., "Why People Fail to Recognize Their Own Incompetence," *Current Directions in Psychological Science*. June 2003; vol. 12 no. 3 83-87.

[vii] G. Riley and J. Lubitz, "Long-Term Trends in Medicare Payments in the Last Year of Life," *Health Services Research*. 2010 April; 45(2): 565–576.

[viii] Of or relating to illness caused by medical examination or treatment.

[ix] http://www.mayo.edu/research/discoverys-edge/uncovering-clues-about-aging-process

[xi] C. Schoen, M.S., R. Osborn, M.B.A., D. Squires, M.M. Doty, Ph.D., R. Pierson, Ph.D., and S. Applebaum, "How Health Insurance Design Affects Access to Care and Costs, by Income, in Eleven Countries," *Health Affairs* Web First, November 18, 2010.

[xii] C. Schoen, R. Osborn, D. Squires, and M.M. Doty, "Access, Affordability, and Insurance Complexity Are Often Worse in the United States Compared to 10 Other Countries," *Health Affairs* Web First, published online Nov. 14, 2013.

[xiii] http://www.pbs.org/newshour/rundown/2012/10/health-costs-how-the-us-compares-with-other-countries.html.

[xiv] Amos Tversky and Daniel Kahneman, "Judgment under Uncertainty: Heuristics and Biases," *Science*, (185) no. 4157. 9/27/1974. Pps 1124-1131.

[xv] J. Temel, J. Greer, A. Muzikansky, E. Gallagher, S. Admane, V. Jackson, C. Dahlin, C. Blinderman, J. Jacobsen, W. Pirl, J. Billings, T. Lynch, "Early Palliative Care for Patients with Metastatic Non-Small-Cell Lung Cancer," *New England Journal of Medicine* 2010; 363:733-742.

[xvi] Shem, *The House of God*, 1978.

[xvii] William T. Vollman, "A Good Death," *Harper's Magazine*, November 2010.

[xviii] Alzheimer's disease accounts for 60-70% of patients with dementia, which refers to a set of symptoms. Other causes of dementia include Lewy body dementia, vascular dementia, Parkinson's disease, depression, and chronic drug use.

[xix] Michael D. Hurd, Ph.D.; Paco Martorell, Ph.D.; Adeline Delavande, Ph.D.; Kathleen J. Mullen, Ph.D.; and Kenneth M. Langa, M.D., Ph.D.; "Monetary Costs of Dementia in the United States," *New England Journal of Medicine*; 368 (April 4, 2013):1326-1334.

[xx] R. Mead, "The Sense of An Ending," *The New Yorker*, May 20, 2013.

[xxi] J.M. Luce and A. Alpers, "Legal aspects of withholding and withdrawing life support from critically ill patient in the United States and providing palliative care to them," *American Journal f Respiratory Critical Care Medicine*, 2000; 162(6):2029-2032.

[xxii] McPhee, S., Winkler, M,: *Care at the Close of Life: Evidence and Experience (JAMA and Archives Journals)*:2011

[xxiii] http://www.acpdecisions.org/about-us/.

[xiv] Alvin C. Kwok, et al., "The Intensity and Variation of Surgical Care at the End of Life: A Retrospective Cohort Study," *The Lancet*, 378:(15 October 2011); pp. 1408 – 1413.

[xxv] "SUPPORT: A controlled trial to improve care for seriously ill hospitalized patients," *JAMA*, 1995;274(20):1591-1598.

[xxvi] "Death With Dignity," *Compassion and Choices* website, May 20, 2013.

# Bibliography

## Books

Adelman, Jeremy. *Worldly Philosopher: The Odyssey of Albert O. Hirschman*. Princeton, NJ: Princeton University Press, 2013.

Barnes, Julian. *Nothing to Be Frightened Of*. New York, NY: Knopf, 2008.

Cain, Susan. *Quiet*. New York, NY: Crown Publishers, 2012.

Cave, Stephen. *Immortality: The Quest to Live Forever and How It Drives Civilization*. New York, NY: Crown Publishers, 2012.

Cohen, Patricia. *In Our Prime*. New York, NY: Simon and Schuster, 2012.

Collins, Billy. *Picnic, Lightning*. Pittsburgh, PA: University of Pittsburgh Press, 1998.

Gray, John. *The Immortalization Commisssion: Science and the Strange Quest to Cheat Death*. New York, NY: Farrar, Straus and Giroux, 2011.

Grimes, Roberta. *The Fun of Dying*. Greater Reality Publications, 2010.

Gutkind, Lee (Editor). *At the End of Life: True Stories About How We Die*. In Fact Books, 2012.

Jacoby, Susan. *Never Say Die: The Myth and Marketing of the New Old Age*. New York, NY: Vintage Books, 2012.

Levy, Alexander. *The Orphaned Adult: Understanding and Coping With Grief and Change After The Death of Our Parents*. Cambridge, MA: Perseus Publishing, 1999.

Kahneman, Daniel. *Thinking, Fast and Slow*. New York, NY: Farrar, Straus and Giroux, 2011.

McAdams, Dan P. *The Redemptive Self: Stories Americans Live By*. New York, NY: Oxford University Press, 2006.

McPhee, Stephen J., Margaret A. Winker, Michael W. Rabow, Steven Z. Pantilat, Amy J. Markowitz, eds. *Care at the Close of Life: Evidence and Experience* (JAMA & Archives Journals). New York, NY: McGraw Hill Medical, 2011.

Nuland, Sherwin B. *How We Die*. New York, NY: Knopf, 1994.

Sharot, Tali. *The Optimism Bias: A Tour of the Irrationally Positive Brain*. New York, NY: Pantheon Books, 2011.

Shem, Samuel. *The House of God*. New York, NY: Dell Books, 1980.

*NHPCO Facts and Figures: Hospice Care in America. National Hospice and Palliative Care Organization* (2009 edition). Alexandria, VA: October 2009.


Newspaper articles


Bernard, Tara Seigel, "The Talk You Didn't Have With Your Parents Could Cost You." *New York Times*, New York, NY. (5/25/2013): B(1).

Brooks, David, "Death and Budgets." *New York Times*, New York, NY. (7/15/2011): A(23).

Carey, Benedict, "This is Your Life (and How You Tell It)." *New York Times*, New York, NY. (5/23/2007): D(1).

Clendinen, Dudley, "The Good Short Life." *New York Times*, New York, NY. (7/10/2011):SR(4).

Ellin, Abby, "A Load Off Their Minds." *New York Times*, New York, NY. (4/23/2013): D(1).

Gross, Jane, "Coming Home For Herbie." New Old Age blog, *New York Times*. July 1, 2008.

Jacoby, Susan, "Taking Responsibility for Death." *New York Times*, New York, NY. (3/31/2012):A(19).

Krieger, Lisa M., "The Cost of Dying: Simple Act of Feeding Poses Painful Choices." www.MercuryNews.Com. Silicon Valley. (11/2/2012).

Leland, John, "In 'Sweetie' and 'Dear,' a Hurt for the Elderly." *New York Times*. New York, NY. (10/6/2008):A(1).

Manheimer, Eric D., "When Doctors Become Patients." *New York Times*, New York, NY. (9/3/2011): A(21).

Marantz Henig, Robin, "A Life-Or-Death Situation." *New York Times*, New York, NY. (7/21/2013):MM(23).

Murphy Paul, Annie, "Your Brain on Fiction." *New York Times*, New York, NY. (3/18/2012):SR(6).

Sacco M.D., Joseph, "At the End of Life, Talk Helps Bridge a Racial Divide." *New York Times*, New York, NY. (8/7/2012):D(5).

Span, Paula, "Among Doctors, A Fierce Reluctance to Let Go." New Old Age blog, *New York Times*, New York, NY. (3/29/2012).

Sullivan, Paul, "Leaving Behind The Digital Keys to Financial Lives." *New York Times*, New York, NY. (5/25/2013): B(7).

Wade, Nicholas, "Prospect of Delaying Aging Ills Is Raised in Cell Study of Mice." *New York Times*, New York, NY. (11/3/2011):A(1,4).

Wilson, Duff, "Conflicts on Health Guideline Panels." *New York Times*, New York, NY. (11/3/2011):B(1,6).

Magazine articles

Banks, James, et al., "Disease and Disadvantage in the United States and in England." *JAMA* 295 (17) (May 3, 2006): 2037-2045.

Block, Susan D., "Helping Patients Make Peace With Death." *Harvard Business Review* (http://blogs.hbr.org/innovations-in-health-care/). (March 8, 2011).

Burkle, Christopher M., et al., "Patient and Doctor Attitudes and Beliefs Concerning Perioperative Do Not Resuscitate Orders: Anesthesiologists' Growing Compliance With Patient Autonomy and Self Determination Guidelines." *BMC Anesthesiology* (online). 2013:13(2)

Chiarella, Tom, "How To Give a Eulogy." *Esquire*. Volume 146, Issue 3. (September 1, 2006).

Cooper, Joshua, et al., "Cardiopulmonary Resuscitation: History, Current Practice, and Future Direction." *Circulation*. Volume 114, (2006): pp. 2839-2849.

Emanuel, Ezekiel, et al., "A Systemic Approach To Containing Health Care Spending." *NEJM*. (September 6, 2012); 367: pp. 949-954.

Emanuel, Ezekiel, et al., "Will Physicians Lead the Way On Controlling Health Care Costs?" *JAMA*. (July 24/31, 2013); 310(4): pp. 374-375.

Ewer, M. S., Kish, S. K., Martin, C. G., Price, K. J. and Feeley, T. W. (2001), "Characteristics of cardiac arrest in cancer patients as a predictor of survival after cardiopulmonary resuscitation." *Cancer*. Volume 92: pp. 1905–1912.

Freed, Janet Carlson (Ed.), "Grief." *Town and Country*. (July 2007): pp. 109-116.

Freedman, David H., "Lies, Damned Lies, and Medical Science." *The Atlantic*. (November 2010).

Gawande, Atul, "Letting Go: What should medicine do when it can't save your life." *The New Yorker*. (August 2, 2010): pp. 38-51.

Gawande, Atul, "The Hot Spotters: Can We Lower Medical Costs By Giving the Neediest Patients Better Care?" *The New Yorker*. (January 24, 2011): pp. 41-51.

Gawande, Atul, "The Way We Age Now." *The New Yorker*. (April 30, 2007): pp. 52-61.

Goodman, Ellen, "Die the Way You Want To." *Harvard Business Review*. (January-February 2012): pp. 58-59.

Hemon, Aleksandar, "The Aquarium: A Child's Isolating Illness." *The New Yorker*. (June 13 & 20, 2011): pp. 50-62.

Hurd, Michael, et al., "Monetary Costs of Dementia in the United States." *The New England Journal Of Medicine*. (April 4, 2013); Volume 368:pp. 1326-1334

Lepore, Jill, "Twilight: Growing old and even older." *The New Yorker*. (March 2, 2011): pp. 30-35.

Kahneman, Daniel, "The Surety of Fools." *New York Times Magazine*. (October 23, 2011): pp. 30-33, 62.

Kane, Jason, "Health Costs: How the U.S. Compares With Other Countries." PBS.org/newshour. (October 22, 2012).

Kutner, J. S., "An 86-year-old woman with cardiac cachexia contemplating the end of her life: review of hospice care." *JAMA*. (January 27, 2010): pp. 349-56.

Kwok, Alvin C., et al., "The Intensity and Variation of Surgical Care at the End of Life: A Retrospective Cohort Study." *The Lancet*, Vol 378:(15 October 2011); pp. 1408—1413.

Luce J. M. and A. Alpers, "Legal Aspects of Withholding and Withdrawing Life Support From Critically Ill Patient in the United States and Providing Palliative Care to Them." *American Journal of Respiratory Critical Care Medicine*. 2000; 162(6):2029-2032.

Marcus, Gary, "Cleaning Up Science." New Desk blog, *The New Yorker*. Posted December 24, 2012.

Mead, Rebecca, "The Sense of an Ending: An Arizona Nursing Home Offers New Ways to Care For People With Dementia." A Reporter At Large (online), *The New Yorker*. Posted May 20, 2013.

Menand, Louis, "Books as Bombs: Why the Women's Movement Needed 'The Feminine Mystique'." *The New Yorker*. (January 24, 2011): pp. 76-79.

O'Rourke, Meghan, "Good Grief: Is There a Better Way To Be Bereaved?" Online, *The New Yorker*. (February 1, 2010)

Peides, Deborah, Arnold Chen, Jennifer, Schore, et al., "Effects of Care Coordination on Hospitalization, Quality of Care, and Health Care Expenditures Among Medicare Beneficiaries: 15 Randomized Trials." *JAMA* (February 11, 2009): pp. 603-618.

Rauch, Jonathan, "How Not to Die." *The Atlantic*. (May 2013): pp. 64-69.

Reisfield G. M., et al., "Survival in cancer patients undergoing in-hospital cardiopulmonary resuscitation: a meta-analysis." *Resuscitation*. 2006, 71(2):pp. 152-160.

Riley, Gerald F., Lubitz, James D., "Long-Term Trends in Medicare Payments in the Last Year of Life." *Health Services Research*. 2010 April; 45(2): 565–576.

Taran, A., et al., "Cardiopulmonary Resuscitation Inpatient Outcomes in Cancer Patients in a Large Community Hospital." *Delaware Medical Journal.* Vol 84, (April 2012):117-21.

Temel, J., et al.. "Early Palliative Care for Patients with Metastatic Non-Small-Cell Lung Caner." *NEJM*. Vol 363, (August 19, 2010): pp. 733-742.

Thompson, MD, PhD, Michael A., "CPR in Advanced Cancer." ASCOconnection.org. March 1, 2013. 10:25 AM.

Tsing Loh, Sandra, "Daddy Issues: Why Caring For My Aging Father Has Me Wishing He Would Die." *The Atlantic.* (March 2012): pp. 84-93.

Volandes, Angelo, et al., "Randomized Controlled Trial of a Video Decision Support Tool for Cardiopulmonary Resuscitation Decision Making in Advanced Cancer." *Journal of Clinical Oncology.* Volume 31, number 3. January 20, 2013: pp. 380-386.

Vollman, William T., "A Good Death: Exit Strategies." *Harper's Magazine.* (November 2010): pp. 36-52.

Winakur, Jerald, "What Are We Going To Do With Dad?" *Health Affairs.* Volume 24. (July 2005): pp. 1064-72.

Woolf, Steven H.; Aron, Laudan; "The US Health Disadvantage Relative to Other High-Income Countries." *JAMA.* (February 27, 2013): pp. 771-2.

"An Array of Errors." *The Economist.* (September 10, 2011): pp. 91-92.

"U.S. Ranks Last Among Seven Countries on Health System Performance Based on Measures of Quality, Efficiency, Access, Equity, and Healthy Lives." The Commonwealth Fund.org/news. (June 23, 2010).

"SUPPORT: A Controlled Trial to Improve Care For Seriously Ill Hospitalized Patients." *JAMA.* 1995;274(20):1591-1598.

About the author

Margaret Overton is the author of the memoir *Good in a Crisis* (Bloomsbury USA). She is also a physician and a mother of two and holds an MFA in Writing from The School of the Art Institute of Chicago.